TRISTIMANIA

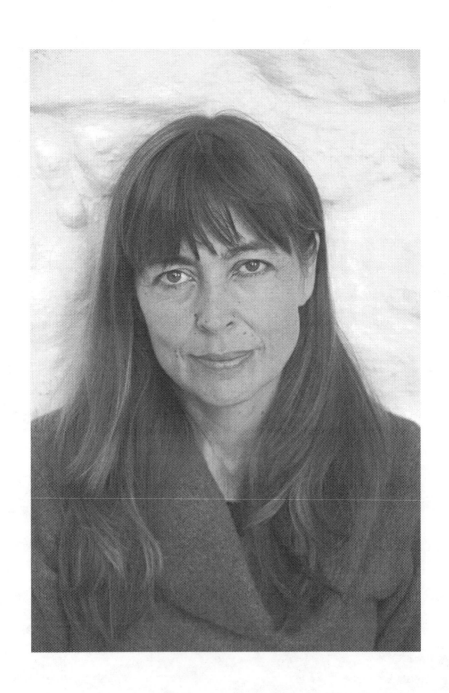

TRISTIMANIA

A DIARY OF MANIC DEPRESSION

JAY GRIFFITHS

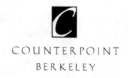

COUNTERPOINT
BERKELEY

Lines on p. 168 from *In Praise of Mortality* by Rainer Maria Rilke, translated
by Anita Barrows and Joanna Macy (New York: Riverhead, 2005), reprinted by
permission of the translators; lines on pp. 177–8 and 184 from *Selected Poems: Rumi*,
translated by Coleman Banks (London: Penguin Books, 2004), copyright © Coleman
Banks, 1995; lines on pp. 97–8 from "Hymn to Hermes" from *Homeric Hymns*,
edited by Nicholas Richardson, translated by Jules Cashford (London:
Penguin Books, 2003), copyright © Jules Cashford, 2003.

Originally published by Hamish Hamilton/Penguin Random House UK

Library of Congress Cataloging-in-Publication Data

Names: Griffiths, Jay, author.
Title: Tristimania : a diary of manic depression / Jay Griffiths.
Description: Berkeley, CA : Counterpoint Press, [2016]
Identifiers: LCCN 2016008987 | ISBN 9781593768
Subjects: LCSH: Manic-depressive illness. | Manic-depressive persons.
Classification: LCC RC516 .G77 2016 | DDC 616.89/5--dc23
LC record available at http://lccn.loc.gov/2016008987
ISBN 978-1-61902-726-8

Cover design by Debbie Berne
Interior design by Jouve (UK), Milton Keynes

COUNTERPOINT
2560 Ninth Street, Suite 318
Berkeley, CA 94710
www.counterpointpress.com

Printed in the United States of America

Paperback ISBN: 978-1-61902-946-0

CONTENTS

PART ONE:
MY MADDEST WEDNESDAY

If I had to pick the moment when it all began, I'd have to choose the afternoon at Twyford Down when I fell down a rabbit hole. Yup, 'strue. So much pain, like lightning striking my ankle, sharp tears smarting in my eyes, the swelling, hobbling clumsy-walking: none of these mattered much. What did matter was that I could not go running and my mind began to fall down its own rabbit holes: it needs to run with serious intent, seeking the self-medication of endorphins, the runner's natural high, leading to the easy tranquillity afterwards.

So, then, I could not run for a month, and something began to go awry in my mind. It was the beginning of a year-long episode of manic depression. For much of the time it would, from the outside, look more like the years left blank in the Medieval Welsh Chronicles as if to say *Nothing Happened This Year*. I did not do any of the things associated with mania and hypomania: I did not have sex with dozens of men; not even one. I did not spend myself into dizzy, indebted oblivion. I did not have any car accidents. Following an earlier episode of hypomania some years before, I'd learnt the pitfalls, so this time I had three rules: no sex, no big spending, no driving – the latter after I had two near-crashes. I sat in my favourite corner of the sofa, nearest to the woodstove. I smoked one rollie after another. Intermittently, I drank too much. End of.

Except it wasn't. The curtain lifted, the veil of the temple of the psyche was rent: I fell through into a further reach of my own mind. The world turned headside out. The interior was made exterior, writ real as plumbing, enormous as opera, jangling with life as if a zoo had eloped with a circus.

According to psychologists, there is an increased risk of manic symptoms in bipolar people at times when they have achieved an important goal, and I was just finishing a book on childhood, *Kith*, which had taken six years of research and writing. I had been working long hours with very little time away from my desk for the previous eighteen months. I was, as one friend said to me, 'writing till the lights go out'. I was burning out, but also, in one of the paradoxes of the mind when it starts to tilt, I was becoming fascinated by the dangerous sparks flickering at the edges of my vision, catching fire and flaming across my mind.

Do episodes of madness have causes? What do they need, to unfurl themselves? They unfold like tragic dramas and, just as tragedy needs a tragic flaw, a backstory and the dramatic incident which kicks off the drama, so chapters of madness also need a tragic flaw (genetic vulnerability), a backstory (long-term stress) and an incident (a trigger).

Genetic vulnerability. Tick.
Long-term stress. Tick.
Trigger? Happened like this.

I'd met a man who was trying to persuade me to work on a project with him. He seemed clever and interesting. We'd gone for a long walk in the hills to talk over the idea. It was a hot day. Halfway up, he wanted to rest and offered me a foot massage. I love foot massages, and I said yes. Foot massage it was, to begin with. I fell into a warm, dreamy state, eyes closed, that deep-relaxation state. And then he wanked all over me.

I would like to tell you that I kicked him in the balls, spat in his face and maybe ironed his nose with a fair-sized rock. I did not. I froze. Like a child in the clutch of a monster, I froze. Like an animal choosing fight, flight or freeze, I froze.

As sexual assault goes, this was mild. Very. But any one-sided sexual encounter is nauseating and utterly humiliating. It left me not just frozen but dazed, bewildered and sick. Soon after he had come, he started saying sorry: he was under no illusion that it was something I wanted – his repeated apologies made that clear. Later, alone, I blamed myself for freezing, for being hopelessly ill-equipped, for 'letting it happen'. I tried to forgive myself. I ran it through in my mind, many times, as if it were a film and I could re-shoot the crucial scene. (Or, indeed, him.) Nothing helped.

In the days after that, I could feel my mind on a slant, every day more off-kilter, every night sleeping less. And then I began to lose my appetite. There are those who comfort-eat, a pal said to me, while there are those who comfort-starve, and this was my pattern. I could not swallow. I could put food in my mouth, but my throat closed up and I had to spit it out.

The clock hands were counting back the hours I could sleep: eight per night, seven, six, five, four, three. Marlowe's Doctor Faustus prays for the hours not to pass: I prayed for them to speed me in sleep. A significant lack of sleep or food (or both) can in itself trigger mentally unstable episodes, and my own genetic predisposition to bipolar disorder or, as I prefer it, manic depression, hurls me to heaven or hell (usually hell) every once in a while. Finishing a book always leaves me vulnerable and exhausted. But in whichever ways one counts the causes, the result was a perfect storm. For three weeks I was in a state of slippage, a gap widening between me and my usual self.

The last time mania had tripped me up, thirteen years previously, I had gone to climb Kilimanjaro, taking my highs to a new height, and then, in the ensuing depression, I had sought help from a shaman in the Amazon who gave me ayahuasca, a profoundly important medicine used in healing for thousands of years. Now, though, there was simply no time.

I knew I had to get to the doctor. I say 'the' doctor because there was only one I'd ever met who I believed could help. He was a local G P. I knew him, and he knew me. I hadn't needed to see him for years, but at the first appointment of this episode, I was crazed with distress. It was not a state bordering on depression but poised on a terrible brink, standing unbalanced and weightless on the rim of a volcano's crater. He didn't hurry me: a ten-minute appointment over-ran to forty minutes and longer, and I was choked with chaos. He offered medication, which I refused initially, but that night I felt worse and made an emergency appointment to see him the following day.

By this time, there was a rupture between what was happening in my mind and what I could say. I couldn't translate myself outwards into the world. I tried to tell him about that terrible disjunction, as if the cabin pressure of my mind were at variance with the pressure of public air. In madness, the head can feel as if it is in a wholly different atmosphere and the consequent psychic pain makes you want to scream.

My doctor contacted the psychiatrist immediately, asking for an urgent appointment. He knew how far and how fast I was falling away from myself and, when he said it was urgent, he meant it.

The following days and nights picked up the reverberations of a sinister percussion, as if my mind were set to an inexorable rhythm, a threatening, ungainsayable, hideous enemy – a drumhead mass, a rhythmic ritual playing me into a deadly war. I felt trapped in a tragedy of terrible teleological intent. Reason was being drummed out into a courtyard to face a firing squad.

In an attempt to feel some kind of control, I tried to chart how mad I felt and put a wavy zigzag line on the pages of my diary, with a note when I first felt my mind slip: November 11th, 'Mercury Goes Awry'. Mercury, god of writers and – surely – god of manic depression (that most mercurial of illnesses), was to play a big part in this strange drama. He flirted with me from the start. I 'heard' (while knowing it was not real) a voice saying: *Meet me at the crossroads.* That, without question, is the voice of Mercury. And his locus. But he is never punctual, and *he* will never wait.

By November 27th my diary has a double wavy line and 'Mercury Double Awry'. By the 29th, my note says 'Mercury Triple Awry' and so it was to stay until January 5th. Months after I'd recovered, I read, with a sense of forceful recognition, the brilliant writer and psychiatrist Kay Redfield Jamison describing the three phases of mania, where stage one is low level, moving to stage two, and then to the third: full-on mania. This is something which may be caught in time – if the professional response is swift.

It wasn't. The psychiatrist's appointment failed to materialize. Instead, the mental health team took a week to respond to the request marked 'urgent' (underlined twice; I saw my doctor's letter), and when they did contact me they offered me an appointment with a psychiatric social worker. *I don't fucking well need a fucking social worker*, I managed not to say. I was ill. They were patronizing. I was furious.

They said they worked as a team. I hated the word 'team' like I hate the word 'family' when it is pronounced, smugly, two syllables, *fam*ly.

Each day was worse than the last.

And then I went mad.

I like the word 'mad', though I prefer its predecessor, *wōd*, of which more later. But 'mad' has its strengths. I like its bluntness; its forthrightness; its very shortness, which brooks no argument. It doesn't bother with sophistication or nuance. It doesn't seek out spectrums of subtlety or gradations of seriousness. Head cleaved open, madstruck.

The root of the word 'mad', from Proto-Germanic, means 'changed (for the worse), abnormal'. Quite. I was changed for the worse. 'I wasn't myself', we say, in that canny phrase.

If there is one part of this episode for which I feel responsible, it was the way I had been seriously overworking and ignoring the warning signs. I'd been pressuring myself to meet difficult deadlines and the stress made my mind gasp in protest. Specifically, I was forcing myself to the gruelling, meticulous, tedious necessity of finishing the index, bibliography and endnotes for *Kith*. It was a carefully researched book, and I couldn't let it out of my hands till all the references and studies were checked. The argument it was presenting (including learning from indigenous cultures) might be unpopular with people who were right-wing or not very bright, but I thought that at least no one would be able to say that each point was not proven, study after study quoted, reference after reference given.

It was the worst kind of work to do when you're ill. Any work would have been too much, but this particular job required conscientious care and neat, whispered referencing, when all the while the howling was in me.

My mind wanted freedom, time and openness; it wanted poetry, wondering-room, sleep, ease and unclocked hours. Instead, it was on a treadmill, no minute spare. The speed with which I was moving was necessary to complete what I'd promised to do before the book went to the printers, and yet that speed itself was contributing to my sense of urgency: the quicker I could finish everything, the sooner I'd have some time off, but the faster I went, the faster this impending crisis was coming, for it was feeding on my speed. I was trying to escape it, even as I was provoking it.

Bricked in, immured, fastened to facts, I felt breathless, panicked and claustrophobic. I was almost fantasizing about the moment when the last detail would be done, when the final footnote had its laces tied, when the last syllable of jot and tittle was bibbed and tuckered, each scruple's weight recorded.

I kept promising myself I'd take a break, a real break, as soon as it was done. But I was too late. The pressure I'd put on myself took its toll. Perhaps if I had followed my own needs and taken a few weeks off, I might have avoided this breakdown.

Instead, every incoming email made me want to scream. If anything was required of me, I felt my bowstring stretched tighter and tighter, bent out of shape, each day tauter. The worse the pressure was, the worse would be the result; I could feel it. When the bow was released, arrow after arrow after arrow would shoot out over my coming days and weeks, injuring and wounding.

I usually work at home but that became impossible. I usually work a full day, but that was suddenly beyond me. For a few days, I forced myself to spend about two hours a day in a shared office-space near me where all the other desks were taken by friends because I thought it would be easier to cope with the screaming in my head. I was using all my willpower to hold the threads, rags and ribbons of my mind together.

I finished what I needed to do, n'er but just. I had to send a couple of emails to turn down offers of work and commissions, the sort of messages one can normally write without a second thought, but the task became a cliff face of impossible reach; it took me hours to gear myself up to do it. My fingers were trembling with the effort to write these excuses, by which I could be excused from my own life.

For one awful moment, I felt the pure panic of an imminent emergency. And then I stopped. My mind staggered, jolted and was sundered. The screen of my mind froze. Time ceased to pass. One intense present moment. Nothing moved. Nothing could move. I could feel no motion in my psyche and all the usual easy fluency of thoughts streaming into each other, confluent and waterful, was slung into reverse. It was the silent onset of sheer dread. It was like the terrible sucking back of the oceans just before a tsunami crashes to the shore; the frightening in-breath before the storm-surge roars inland. The sky was going to fall through the sea, the clouds would smash on impact like glass, and the great pale sheet of a dead white sky, motionless, frozen and broken, would lie noiseless at the bottom of the ocean.

But the ocean was in the wrong place. So was the sky. And the shore. Nothing was speaking as it should. The horses were stampeding to higher ground. The gulls fled in fear; all the birds were in silent flight. The water was milling, a mob-anger moving it. The wave was crossing the oceans towards me. Later, I knew, would come the disaster, the broken houses and crushed cars, the lamp-posts bent in two. Now was only now, stark and brutal.

I was staring at the computer screen, and I think I said, 'Fuck!' a couple of times, in a whimper of fear. One of my friends turned to me.

– Are you okay? she asked seriously, nervously almost.

– I've. Got. To. Go. Home.

I pulled these words out of memory, as if I were speaking a foreign language unused for years, each word needing utter concentration. And I fled home, like a terrified animal seeking the safest place it knows. I tried desperately not to meet anyone's eyes, wishing I could be invisible, finding the two hundred yards an almost unconquerable distance. I felt my terror must be visible on my face, as if my mind had stepped outside my skull, white and frozen.

My mind! I've broken it! was all I could think. It was blank: deadly blank. After the fire, after the flood, after the bomb, after the tsunami. As I got to my front door, I tried to use logic: *This cannot be happening because it has never happened before.* Useless. My exclamation turned to pleading: *This must not happen.* The last clear thing I remember is being on all fours in my study, my hands hammering the floor, saying aloud to myself over and over again: *I am losing my mind. I am losing my mind. I am losing my mind.*

For the next twelve hours I was in a kind of delirium. I was giggling one moment then crying; soaring then crashing. My moods were swinging within minutes, flinging me from the thrilling high-wire paradise of exuberance to the wrenching agony of a pain so gripping I could hardly breathe. It was a Wednesday, my maddest Wednesday, *mercredi* in French, the day of Mercury indeed.

I was hallucinating, and I could see spirals rising, each one spinning upwards faster and faster the more I watched it, like the tiny flecks you can see with your eyes shut which fall faster if you follow them with your gaze.

Some medical conditions can be called 'florid' and it is a particularly apt term for mania, the sick psyche's self-flowering, *les fleurs du* very very *mal*. I could see unreal blooms – the idea of flowering without the actual flowers, wandering bloomings, the very blossom of the mind – a rose arose, blossomed and bloomed and was blown. Then my hallucinations turned to blood and silence. I lost my words. I could think only in images. In the small hours of the night, I sat by my woodstove and got the giggles because I found the woodstove so comical a companion. One of my cats crept near me, and I cried in pity for its languageless state. Even as I was myself.

'Tristimania' is an old term for manic depression, precisely capturing that sense of grief and hilarity, of violent sadness and mad highs. I tried to go to bed, but my pillows made me laugh. Eventually, I fell asleep, but I woke within the hour to find my pillow soaked with tears, as I had been crying in my sleep. Tristimania in an hour.

Set free of all ties to Earth, sense and gravity, I achieved escape velocity. I woke, if that's the word, to a weird waking dream, a flight of fire towards whatever burns, burning on the inside, in an incandescence of the mind and mad – out – out – to somewhere so beyond Earth it felt like I was circling with the moons of Jupiter, for circles appeal to the cycling mind. Jupiter is jovial, Jove, bringer of jollity, and that thought made me gleeful, particularly because its moon is Puck, the Trickster of the skies, a fellow mad and manic moon who, when I began to fall, slipped away laughing.

There are galaxies within the human mind, and madness wants to risk everything for the daring flight, reckless and beautiful and crazed. Everyone knows Icarus fell. But I love him for the fact that he dared to fly. Mania unfurls the invitation to fly too high, too near the sun, which will melt the wax of the mind, and the fall will be terrible.

Then I saw my wings. They were of a piece with this mad reverie: they were like a field of stars in a midnight sky. It seemed obvious that I had wings, because we all do: wings of mind. The previous time I'd had an episode of hypomania, I had spent a lot of time with one particular friend. I always knew he was an angel, but I had suddenly seen his wings and they were white, plump, pillowy, deep with downy feathers, as pure and healing as sleep.

How real did I think they were, these wings? True, but not actual. Not literally, palpably present, but still a profound truth of the mind.

It is wise to be amphibious, to swim between the world of metaphor and of reality, but, increasingly, I was reality's orphan and the inhabited world was dead for me because I was alive only to dream, poetry, messengers and metaphors. Metaphor was a prism surrounding me: real light entered and irreal rainbows resulted. Poetry and reality had swapped densities: poetry mattered more, and had more intense mattering, than the unsure real.

In all those mad hours, I could only 'see' one sane thing. In my hallucinations, I could see one little, thin silver thread – of lucidity – twirling like a lifeline from the moons of Jupiter through the terrifying spaces between the stars and down to the Earth, exactly to my doctor's surgery. As my psyche careered unsecured, veering and circling and boundless, this was the only time in twelve hours that I had access to words in my mind, to just one verbal thought: 'I seem to have forgotten my parachute. I must ask Dr Leslie if he has one.'

Overall, if one feeling overrode all the others, it was terror. I am not often fearful, and I've also tried to do things even when they do scare me. Some years earlier, I had gone alone to West Papua, to write about the ongoing genocide there. Writers and journalists are forbidden entry, and the invading Indonesians have shot people for reporting on the situation. I was decently frightened but I also felt distressed and angry about the way Indonesia seemed able to bully the world into silence. I had bought a plane ticket, put 'tourist' in the box marked 'reason for visit' and gone. It was frightening, for sure, but not as frightening as going mad.

Schumann wrote to his wife, Clara, of the night between 17th and 18th October 1833: 'I was seized with the worst fear a man can have, the worst punishment Heaven can inflict – the fear of losing one's reason . . . Terror drove me from place to place. My breath failed me as I pictured my brain paralysed. Ah, Clara, no one knows the suffering, the sickness, the despair, except those so crushed.'

The horses of reason were being attacked by the tigers of madness, terror and shock the results. I was frightened partly because I did not know who could protect me if I couldn't protect myself, but, of itself, going mad is terrifying. To be more precise, it is intermittently terrifying and the fear hits you in the moments of lucidity when you glimpse yourself in the wayward mirror and see yourself in a shaft of real light.

'Lucid': an anagram of 'ludic'. In the free play of my ludic mind, the lucid moments were seriously sobering. The ludic times were an exuberant delight, mind on helium, ballooning skywards, bouncing in rubber clouds of unknowingness. I collected the moments of lucidity in which I realized I was going mad. Carefully, I wrote them down, ludicity recollected in lucidity. I clung to these fragments of self-knowing.

At about noon the following day, I had one such moment of lucidity. I tried to phone the doctors but my voice was cracking open and I was scared I would scream. Perhaps the intensity of a mad person's speech is partly due to the effort it takes not to scream, or roar or groan or let out the unworded wound-noises of an animal in pain. The surgery is – luckily – close to my house, so I walked in. In the waiting room, I could feel the normalcy of others circulating like a common cold, and the sheer ordinariness was calming. I had been rehearsing my lines:

– Please can I make an appointment with Dr Leslie?

I was forcing myself to keep my voice level, and trying not to forget how to say this. It's incredible to me, looking back, quite how hard that was. Just nine words. A path over a precipice, with gulfs of screaming chaos on either side. Nine words to get me across.

There was no available appointment for days. I took a deep breath and said very quietly and slowly and urgently:

– I–need–to–see–him.

My thought processes had been kidnapped. Each word was like a hostage of meaning smuggled out under the kidnapper's nose.

– You can see another doctor, the receptionist said gently.

I took a deep breath.

– He–told–me–to–get–a–message–to–him–if–I–needed–to.

If I couldn't see him, I knew I was at the end of something. I thought I might convulse like a fish out of water, a hideous grotesquerie of a physical performance of this mental floundering, drowning in air.

– He's doing an emergency surgery this afternoon. You could come back at four.

Saved.

Then it was a matter of holding the molecules of the self together for four hours. A friend had planned to come by. He took me for a short drive, just for something to do other than sit on the sofa trying not to jabber. But though he drove carefully and slowly, the motion and speed of the car made me vertiginously anxious, like a shriek of sawn nerves, and we had to turn back.

Four o'clock came. I nearly fell into the doctor's office. He was shocked that in a week the mental health team had failed to give me an appointment. He would, he said, have felt happier with a psychiatrist's diagnosis, but he would have to make decisions on his own. To him, it looked like mixed-state hypomania, and slipping worse: hallucinations mean you're entering psychotic territory. He said he'd phone the psychiatrist so at the very least he could get confirmation of the antipsychotic medication he was proposing.

– Whatever it is, I want a low dose, I managed to say.

I felt as if I were not speaking my thoughts but rather dredging up a memory of what 'I', the un-mad person, would have wanted to say. I was frightened of the idea of antipsychotic medication, particularly as I'd seen a brilliant friend of mine sectioned for a manic episode and given so much lithium that he became a slur-mountain of shambling zombieness. There was little left of him, and it took him years to recover from the medication. It was as if I were appealing to the slip of logic that threaded my mind, as if I were asking my memory of myself to take power of attorney over my current threadbare, madswept self.

The doctor told me to go home and wait by the phone, and he'd call me when he had spoken to the psychiatrist.

– Can I check we have the right phone number for you? he asked.

I said nothing.

– What's your phone number?

This was it.

I could not remember it.

Chasm.

This was the hardest question I'd ever been asked in my life. My mind shut down every other activity in order to focus on it, because of what the inability to answer would mean. Gone. Sunk. Drowned. Sanity is to the psyche what oxygen is to the body; its loss, even momentary, hits the mind shockingly because it is speaking the language of ultimates: life and death. My mind was losing its oxygenating sanity. It was as if Dr Leslie had asked the question from miles away, from a shore whose safety I could not reach. I wanted to say 'Help', but even that word was a luxury in the drowning mind's innerness, its internal compression of need to an absolute imperative, beyond help, beyond calling.

How brief a moment it probably was in real-time but how long a moment in psyche-time. How invisible to an observer this moment would have been and yet the enormity of the drama within me. My fear muted me into unobservable panic, a shut-down, a white-out. I can remember this now, as if it happened an hour ago. The psyche will fight for its life, reckless of anything beyond itself. I felt the ferocity of the need, the almost physical sense of raging emergency, and I knew I would ruthlessly fight, struggle or latch on to anything in order not to drown.

And then I felt as if my mind split into two: the drowning mind which simply couldn't remember and the watching mind which saw truly the gravity of the situation. I was down to the fundamentals of the psyche. Everything else had spooled away, the lovely skeins of linking things; thoughts, words, feelings, selfhood or relationships were not in fact the centre. At the real centre was an instinct to survive. Something I'd call core mind. Ferocious. Adamantine. In the bitten vehemence of the violent need to survive, I was at the cold, hard kernel of implacable willpower. My psyche was down to its bones, down to the bleached calcium of a revenant star, the obdurate bones of the psyche, which are harder than iron or steel, harder than the hexagonal diamond, the hardest mineral on earth.

I never did answer the question. Instead my doctor read out to me the phone number he had and asked me if I recognized it. I didn't. He read it out more slowly, and I did.

He moved fast, sending me home, getting hold of the psychiatrist, confirming the medication, calling me back in, all in minutes. He agreed to start on a low dose and had one of the pills in his hand to show me how to halve it. I wanted to take the one he was holding in his fingers, in a kind of sympathetic magic. I have always loved the placebo effect, and I thought the medication would work better if I had this particular pill. It combined magical thinking with the logic of placebo studies. I have never taken a pill so quickly. Thanks to that, things were about to get better. And worse.

The pill was fast-acting. My friend took me out to a place where he could have dinner and I could try to. Three hours after I'd taken the pill I could swallow, and I ate half a veggie burger and some chips; more than I'd eaten in days. That night, I slept for six hours, twice the amount I had been sleeping for some time. When I woke, I went downstairs to where my friend was sleeping on the sofa and I sat near him and held his hand for hours.

The next day, I got the psychiatrist's appointment. While I was in the waiting room, the social worker asked if she could come along into the appointment. *I'm not a fucking sideshow*, I thought and bit back. Do these people not realize how hard it is to deal with even *one* stranger when you've gone mad? The psychiatrist was late back from his lunch and seemed flippant about it. I followed him into his office, watching his feet. He wore winklepickers, which I disliked intensely. My initial loathing was confirmed in seconds. His questions sounded to me like something you'd find in a pop-psychology quiz in *Cosmo*. I felt he was trying to catch me out in self-contradictions, and it was like being interrogated by P C Plod, oafishly trying to outwit someone who has committed no crime. He sat trapping my words in lumping handwriting. I made myself un-approachable: I think he wrote that I had a problem with authority. He seemed to think of psychiatric illness purely as a brain malfunction, a mechanical problem. To me, the psyche is also a matter of the soul.

But knowing I was mad, and not feeling any trust in the psychiatrist, I felt I must tread a delicate path, giving him enough information so that he could give an accurate diagnosis but without providing any reason for high-dose medication or any excuse to section me. I was judging how little I could get away with saying, while ensuring that I said enough. I was concentrating all my attention on this, like taking an exam on which my life depended. This was made worse because part of my mind knew I'd gone mad, so I was in a logical predicament: I knew my judgement was untrustworthy and yet I knew I had to trust my instinct for who could help me and who couldn't. He may well have been trustworthy – indeed, he may well have been a perfectly good psychiatrist – but the point was whether or not I could find it in myself to trust. And I could not. My intuition would have to compensate for my lack of judgement.

There were also things I didn't feel like saying, out of a sense of privacy, almost of decorum. The previous time I'd had an episode of hypomania, thirteen years earlier, I had slept with eight different men over a couple of weeks. It was a kind of sexual larceny against my usual monogamous instinct. The emotional aftershocks of that particular self-spending spree were, well, *rather awkward*. But when the psychiatrist asked about previous episodes, specifically angling for answers to do with unwise and intemperate sexual encounters, although I knew that was one of the tell-tale signs of mania and hypomania, I refused to answer.

In any case, for me, the acting out of hypomania was uninteresting; it was a way of literalizing a profoundly metaphoric experience, and this time around I wanted to explore the manic world for its metaphors. I certainly felt that lovely hot purring of sexuality from time to time – especially when one of my friends, playing Nogood Boyo, was flirting with me outrageously – but actually having sex seemed both too dangerous and far too literal. If I physically acted out these invitations, it would have felt crude, the mind miming its metaphors in the clowning body; rather, I wanted to let my psyche explore its non-literal and far subtler landscapes.

Shakespeare's clown, Will Kemp, in what he called his 'nine days wonder', morris-danced from London to Norwich, and that seems to me something which could appeal only to the manic-minded, for the flaring energy of mania craves expenditure. While the need to spend your entire body's energy is acknowledged in the literature, it seems unlikely to be a priority in diagnostic questioning. Manic 'spending' is often enacted in the form of money, and this seems to be a narrow focus of psychiatric questions. Those enquiries also lean heavily on whether a patient has been 'spending' themselves sexually, perhaps because our society is obsessed with the crudely countable: it is easier to ask patients how much money they've spent or how many people they've slept with than to ask if they've skipped with the electric jubilation of a six-year-old or to attempt to measure the vastness of their love for the universe.

When my doctor saw the report from the psychiatrist, he was glad his diagnosis had been seconded and told me that, reading between the lines, the appointment had not been wholly successful.

– It's okay. We'll look after you here, I remember him saying.

I wanted to weep with relief.

Memory goes odd in madness: some conversations, events and mental happenings are etched unforgettably in my mind. Other moments, though, are wholly void: blanks of memory which I know are blanks only because my friends have sometimes asked me if I remember a certain thing, and the occasional total memory failure makes me poignantly embarrassed. A friend had phoned me in the epicentre of this madness and asked how I was. I apparently answered with a kind of gleeful clarity, 'I am in the middle of a spec-TAC-ular breakdown,' and started giggling manically. I had forgotten that completely until he reminded me, months later.

A few things, meanwhile, are self-evidently misremembered. I was half convinced that an early appointment with my doctor had been in the corridor of the surgery, because I was then puta-tively halfway between being in his care and in the care of the psychiatrist. My mind was waywardly transposing emotional truth to actual fact, and I found myself imploring my trust in my own logic and in my doctor. Number one: I knew he wouldn't have fixed an appointment in the corridor. Number two: I knew I was mad. Therefore this was not a real memory but a hallucinatory one. How precious reason is, when one is losing one's mind. This was the first of many times when I had an implacable, ferocious sense of clinging to logic – pure, almost mathematically logical steps of thinking – in order not to drown in the mind's expansive, oceanic imaginings, although the siren voices cried to me to lose myself in the wildest waters.

And I – drowning.

My mind couldn't hold itself together; it couldn't carry its own weight. I tried to hold on to anything that could give me compre-hension and coherence. I read the leaflets about my medication obsessively, as if the words spelling out their curative power were also healing spells. I sometimes sought in the language of science the descriptions of the structures of the mind, though I could barely concentrate for more than a few sentences. Often, I found that when I turned the dial in my mind, there was nothing except static hum, the sound of furry electricity, but if I could tune into someone else, I could borrow their sense and sensibleness. I often phoned friends briefly, just to hear language being broadcast on the frequency of sanity.

I began trying to write down what I felt in the moments when I was collected enough, because the written words anchored me and gave me a sense of safety, as if a line of words across the page were a lifeline. Words were a slender thread to logic, which was a stronger rope to lucidity. I was desperate for something of *logos* which the sick and careering drowner in the illogical, hallucinatory, voluptuously mad psyche could hold to. Tough. Taut. Rope. Often I wrote down the same thing many times, forgetting I'd remembered it already. These shards I took to friends and to doctor's appointments in case, otherwise, I would turn up, sit down and be speechless. With these shards, I could give them fragments of sense about the madness which engulfed me.

I never lost my insight, according to my doctor; never lost the overseeing part of the mind which charts the craziness of the other parts. Sometimes I had to use all my willpower and all the sternness of logic to support this insight. I wanted neither to overstate nor understate my psychological condition, and this accuracy seemed vital for two reasons. The first was medical, so that my doctor could assess medication and dosage, because the fluctuating nature of these episodes means that medication must also be fluctuating; alterations must be tailored as closely as possible to needs and moods which are ever-changing. The second was a strong sense of the abstract relationship between truth and wellness. The truth will heal; lies will kill.

My notebooks have always been very precious to me and I travel with them wrapped, waterproofed, closer to me than my passport or money. They are footprints of my thoughts, tracks of journeys, curiosity-paths and desire-lines. I have never surrendered my notebooks to anyone to hold except once, in the Amazon, crossing difficult rivers on rickety bridges, when there was a real risk I'd lose my footing, so I gave my notebooks to my guides for safekeeping because their balance was surer than mine. Now, I felt I was giving not my notebooks but my psyche itself to my doctor for safekeeping – *please can you carry my mind for a while?* – because I'd lost my mental balance. I was scared I'd drop my psyche in this torrent, frightened I'd lose my mind downstream, but I knew he could hold it safe and give it back to me when I was able to look after it myself again.

I tried to spend time outside, and I was managing to run again. One morning I saw a robin singing in a high branch, and the angle of its beak was the angle of hope: those extra degrees beyond the necessary and the abundance of bird-joy and robin-poetry made me cry for its song of well-being. The sheer goodness of nature for the sick psyche is incomparable; there in green one is not judged, one is accepted, with consolation and company. Nature gives you the exalted, tender ordinary – as of right.

'Buy lemon drizzle cake for Ann,' it says in my diary on one of those early days. It is the kind of jotted reminder of a day-to-day, welcome task of friendship. These utterly ordinary plans, undemanding and easy, become to the disordered mind something like an impossible quest, a fight with Grendel's mother or the giant on the bridge. I had to blow on the palms of my hands, let my mind take a warrior stance, as the job of leaving the house and buying a lemon drizzle cake was like engaging in mortal combat. It was the same with Christmas tasks: organizing presents for my nephews and godchildren had an immensity and implacable necessity which made me feel sick with dread. Looking back, I at first could not understand why I didn't just say to myself and others: *Sorry, guys, I'm not well.* The tasks became vitally important to perform because not being able to do even the simplest of things is a measure of how low you're scoring in the competence stakes, proof-brutal that what you fear is true. You are mad. You can't cope.

For the same reason, I did housework doggedly, with white-faced intent, as if my life depended on it. Psychoanalyst and author Darian Leader notes, in his superb book on the precise motifs of manic depression, *Strictly Bipolar*, that one feature of manic depression is 'the ubiquitous obsessive phenomena of tidying and ordering' and, for myself, if I could see myself functioning in the most basic of ways – the washing-up done, my socks clean – then I could imagine I was keeping madness at bay, at least in its visible signs. Dirt was the evidence of non-functioning. Cleaning would hold back the signs of madness. It would wipe away the tell-tale fingerprints of insanity. Of housework, Leader writes: 'It would be difficult to find a case of manic-depression where this activity does not have an important place . . . it [is] a way of creating an elementary binary, of separating good and bad, dirty and clean.' I was grateful to read this, because it was so precisely my experience; a bipolarity not just of temperament but of categorizing. It is common knowledge that one's emotions – agony or ecstasy – tend to polarities, but one's *ideas* seek polarity, too. Devils and angels, or hell and heaven, seem like ideas created by a manic-depressive divinity. Black and white as a piano keyboard.

The piano keyboard itself was a key image, if you'll excuse the pun. I play the piano and, at this point in my madness, I saw the mind like a piano, where the range goes from the lowest bass notes of grief, rising towards sadness, then the ordinary reticulation of difficulties, then up into tranquillity, further up to happiness and – tops – an ode to pure joy in the treble notes. But manic depression plays the mind an extra trick. It is as if depression is an invisible and inaudible octave below the lowest notes on a keyboard and mania is an invisible and inaudible octave above. The mad mind, playing in the ranges inaudible to others, is only too audible to itself, and in mixed states the resonances of the highest notes appeal to the lowest, which in turn hurl the sweeping arpeggios straight back up again.

As well as the antipsychotic, I was also taking a mood stabilizer, Depakote. I was grateful, and they were certainly effective: if my mind was a small boat in stormy waters, it felt as if the anti-psychotic stopped the boat rising and falling while Depakote calmed the sea itself. But I hated taking them. Why would you ever want to dampen this incandescence? How could you allow your flight-feathers to be trimmed? Obviously, my friends said, because you will crash, and the crashes are dreadful; that is what you are medicating. But mania cannot recall depression, as drunkenness cannot recall hangovers – and as depression, in its own way, cannot recall ordinary happiness.

During these days I received an email from a friend of mine who is an author and psychiatrist, asking how I was. I kept it brief, describing this episode, and I think I mentioned wings. 'Angels are present but the destroying angel is also there,' he wrote back, in a sobering message. (Rilke called angels the 'almost deadly birds of the soul'.) More than anything, he urged me over and over to take all the prescribed medication. This was hard.

When I had the appointment with the psychiatrist, he had told me that Depakote wasn't something he'd prescribe for women of childbearing years but that it was fine for someone like me, who hadn't wanted children. To me, his remarks seemed off-hand and presumptuous, and I felt hurt. I had dearly wanted a child and, in all my depression, this was an unquenchable sadness. Every time I'd taken the Depakote pills, I had thought of the psychiatrist, and that made me detest the medication even more. Putting those pills in my mouth was like swallowing his words. I told my doctor this, and from then on he used a good-natured sleight of hand, mentioning that the generic name for Depakote was 'sodium valproate', a term which did not have negative associations for me. So he simply persuaded me to take sodium valproate. I don't know if he consciously did that or whether his easy instinct for persuasion supplied the ruse under his own radar. But it worked. I let myself be persuaded by the feint and involved myself in a willing suspension of backchat.

Meanwhile, my psychiatrist friend made himself available by email and I leant on his sagacity. His first career was in English literature, but then he had retrained as a doctor and psychiatrist. From one discipline, he understood the individual mind, co-influent with world-mind in poetry and music, and from the second he knew the necessity to take medication as a matter of life and death.

It is well known that people with bipolar disorder are often not 'compliant' with medication. This is a dreadful term to use. While it may be spoken with a precise and simple medical meaning (i.e.

someone not taking prescribed meds), it is heard in its general lay meaning: someone being obedient, conforming, trying to please, fitting into the system. Although manic depression has some shared motifs, yet the experience of it can also be flamboyantly idiosyncratic, and those in the middle of an episode are indeed the opposite of a compliant character.

Also, simply, we're having far too much fun: in one's own head there are fireworks and firewords, high-wire acts and high-wired arts, ecstatic stars in a precession of delirious hilarity; a party, an opera, an explosion of exuberance. Why on earth would you want to come back down?

It was obviously wise to take medication, but mania – or, possibly, one could say the manic personality – loves a dare, is seduced by audacity. Risk winks broadly. Boldness allures. That daredevil mania is compelling: it is ravishing and beguiling, licking its lovely, illicit lips to invite you to play.

Meanwhile, the integrity of the self feels compromised on pills. Taking antidepressants, I can feel like a puppet on a string: the higher the dose, the more I dance; the lower the dose, the more I collapse. Taking antipsychotics and mood stabilizers was oddly humiliating: I was flattened and numbed by something outside myself.

Where does self end and illness begin? Is manic depression a quintessential part of oneself, or quite the opposite: an illness which skews you to its own image? Does the medication alter who you are? Does one become inauthentic in taking these mind-altering substances? Is it 'natural' – that heavily contested word – to take drugs like these?

Usually, we think of our 'self' as including both body and mind, and not one without the other. But my mind was a runaway in mania, and a stowaway in depression: either way, not fully present, even while my body was providing its alibi: Look, I am still here: see my hands (although they are unguided), see my feet (although they are undirected).

A friend of mine, a philosopher keen on questions of selfhood, asked if manic depression felt like my self or like something external taking over, like being possessed by something. It's something which concerns me. If you take bipolarity away from one's sense of identity, what else must you take away? One's artistic ability? Temperament? Sensibility? Empathy? Capacity for friendship and communication? To me, the experience of having had manic depression can never be separated from my sense of who I am. It runs through me like wine through water: everything is coloured (or tainted) by it. Most of the time, I feel as if the self is semi-permeable and can, up to a point, take in elements of the outer world and yet keep its selfhood intact, like drinking alcohol, so alcohol is outside the self and, once consumed, the expression of intoxication is one's own. But this is true only up to a point, beyond which one drunk person seems much like another; similarly, at the extreme of depression, one deeply depressed person is very like another, the symptoms outshouting the individual. In depression, I feel I have been taken over and have lost my self entirely. Instead, a rude incumbent has slumped into my life, leaving half-eaten sarnies under the sofa and stale smells in every room.

Further questions arise: if manic depression has a signature, recognized between 'sufferers', then that signature is not part of an individual's discrete identity. It gives every sufferer a similar script, even though that script is enacted and accented very differently by each individual. Perhaps, then, it might be more accurate to think of manic depression less as a part of the individual mind than part of 'world-mind', which wants to communicate, to speak, to step over boundaries between self and self, not just between one 'sufferer' and another but beyond, outwards, to branch out like art in all its mani-fold forms, to speak, link and connect mind to mind. Darian Leader's work on the signatures of manic depression includes the 'sense of connectedness with other people and with the world . . . The exhil-aration that the sense of connectedness brings must be communi-cated . . . [in an] unquenchable thirst for an addressee'. He quotes Terri Cheney, manic depressive and author, writing: 'manic sex isn't really intercourse. It's discourse, just another way to ease the insati-able need for contact and communication.'

Is manic depression even an illness? One definition of illness is that it impairs normal functioning, but in the foothills of mania normal functioning is enhanced. If 'illness' is something unwanted, then manic depression is certainly not always an illness: if I medi-cated myself to median, middle C, all the time, I would miss myself. If I didn't have this condition at all, I would miss a world. This is a very common response in people with bipolar disorder, as Stephen Fry illustrated in his documentary *The Secret Life of the Manic Depressive*, when he asked each contributor whether, given the chance, they would press a button to rid themselves of the condition. All but one said they would not.

Manic depression is both artist and assassin. While it plays artist, it is on your side: generous, generating, connective and vital. But then the psychomachy begins, a battle between a God and a Devil for the possession of the soul, and the artist stealthily becomes assas-sin. In depression, the mind feeds on itself, self-cannibalizing. The soul-loss of depression is well attested, and many people in the anguish of depression know that familiar cry: 'I hate my self.' At this point, when it is destroying, deathful and endangering mind and life, it no longer feels like 'me'. The changeover happens incrementally, like gatecrashers arriving one by one at a party until there are more gatecrashers than friends. It is no longer your party. The house is ransacked, the food truffled up, the wine drunk.

I had snatches of competence when I could read emails and reply, but these moments were unreliable. If there was a little clearing in the cloud, I'd send and receive, then my mind greyed over again. My writer friends wrote me messages which acted like spells: one wrote to say, 'I feel as if I am standing next to you, holding hands wordlessly, watching the holiness together.' Another sent me intelligent and wise comfort many times over the worst months, and the hugs of an armoured bear. But no one – no one – can walk with you in the landscape of nightmare.

Nightmare is a realm sadistically tailored to your own psyche; bad enough when you're well. But when I was sick and insomniac, the few hours of sleep I had were Mafia-attacks, boiled heads with grotesque and fearful brutalities, as if Hieronymus Bosch were twisting day thoughts to night terrors. In one, I was stabbed by a misogynist mob, and then I had to watch a writer friend being crucified; I was helpless as he hung by his wrists on meat hooks.

A friend and I went to the sea one day, and every encounter seemed freighted with enormity; a flock of starlings swooped over us in their hundreds, and I felt the rush of wings like the breath of a God I do not believe in. There was a makeshift shrine tucked into the cliff, dedicated to 'Our Lady of Craig Lais', with stone circles and mosaics, spangly scarves, candles, feathers, ribbons, painted rocks, joss sticks and gorse petals. This was how my mind felt, as if its wholeness were fractured in mosaics of starlight at the cliff edge of feeling; as if my mind were perched on the windswept shrine, a feather for every wind, sometimes dazzled by the brightness and brilliance of the world and then – all is chiaroscuro – demented by the dark rocks of cliff caves where the deep water hurled itself to hurt.

Mixed-state hypomanic episodes affect the mind's sight; one moment you cannot see because you are blinded with light and the next because you are blinded with darkness. A midwinter scene gashed with light: blackness of an eclipsed sun in midsummer. It may be midnight at noon, or noon at midnight, but the light flips twofold so light is always darkening and dark always lightening, in the two-light or twi-light of the mind.

The intensity of both the highs and the lows altered time, so each day felt like a week in its passing, while if I glanced backwards a month had gathered its meanings and stories and was a life's journey. In manic-time, one travels at high speed while everyone else seems to be going very slowly in comparison. Accordingly, when you're racing and over-capable and wildly energetic, any ordinary human speed looks like lethargy and feeds, I think, the irritability which many people feel in mania and hypomania. This speed is part of mania's hyper-connectedness, because the manic mind wants to connect everything in a flash; it wants instantaneity, a fabulous explosion of nowness.

In depression, time is disconnected from the time of others. The schedules don't fit. Everyone else is going too fast. Days sag without spine or recognizable time. No nature, no time passing, no verbs. Art has its face to the wall. Fresh food is stale by the time it is on the plate. There are fruit flies like baboons. You'd need the strength of Atlas to bear it. You have the strength of a sick kitten.

Depression can have its own awful now, when the anguish of a lifetime seems to be felt in the aggregate, as if time is not linear – nothing has passed, nothing is over – but as if everything is hideous with intensity so even the future seems to fold backwards and lean its illimitable, impossible weight on this moment. In depressed hours, all the times of my life pooled in me and all my past was black water circling inexorably, bearing down on me, in a whirlpool, a gyre of centripetal pain.

Depression is a Black Hole consuming time, both containing it and negating it. The graveness of depression feels like 'gravity's relentless pull', as scientists describe a Black Hole. It sucks an entire human life into itself; nothing can withstand its pitiless tug into sheer black nothingness, a force field of pure negativity. In what is called 'gravitational time dilation', an object falling into a Black Hole appears to slow down as it approaches the event horizon, taking an infinite time to reach it. At the centre of a Black Hole is a 'gravitational singularity'. In the depressed psyche, everything relates – singularly – only to itself. The deadly disconnection. The closer the psyche steps towards the event horizon, the closer it is to being sucked in. Nothing, not even light, can escape from inside. Wholly hollow, yet containing everything that was once a life, depression is a hideous anti-pregnancy, a gross reabsorption of life, a swallowing of vitality so nothing is born or can be. No light, no life, no joy.

What does 'psychotic' mean?

There are some words (and this is one) whose very definitions seem to depend on their being applied to other people. 'Psychopath', 'murderer', 'sadist', 'psychotic': Other, they suggest. Terrifying and inexplicable.

Since I was at this point taking antipsychotics, I could (and had to) assume it might mean I was psychotic. I, not Other. And not terrifying either, since even in my deepest madness I was unaggressive. Was the word inexplicable? Is there ever a word you cannot gently hold in your hand, smoothing out its folds like the frown line on your own forehead, and in it find – aha! the clarity – the explicated? I took out my dictionary. I looked up the definition. I saw that 'psychotic' meant suffering a severe mental derangement, especially when resulting in delusions and loss of contact with external reality. I could see it was quite reasonably applied to me, since I had been hallucinating.

I put away my dictionary.

I am psychotic.

Impossible.

I took out the dictionary again, like revisiting a dauntless friend who will keep telling you the truth you need to hear.

The definition fits.

I put the dictionary away again.

I am psychotic.

Impossible.

Begin again, Michael Finnegan, begin again.

Beckettian.

I could understand psychosis better if I cast my nets otherwise, so I found out more about the antipsychotic I was taking, and read that it worked for psychosis by correcting the balance of the neurotransmitters, the chemicals that control the function of nerve pathways in the brain. The message system had gone awry. The terrain of the tricksy messenger. For in those nets I cast, I pulled in that lovely quicksilver fish: Mercury or Hermes, the messenger, Trickster of the ancient pantheon. The brain's heft and weight were toys in his hands: careless with gravity, feckless with the import of things, turning weight to slightness, Mercury was playing tiddlywinks with my sanity.

PART TWO:
THE CONDITION OF PASSION

— Why write about that terrible year? a friend of mine asked me recently. How can you want to revisit it?

— Why would you climb the mountains of the mind? Because they are there, my friend, because they are there.

Because manic depression seduces, like mountains do, and kills, as they do. Because, too, it is survivable with skilful help.

Because this condition can be seen as a form of illness, but it is not only an illness; it also hurls the mind into a world of metaphor, and to regard it solely as a medical issue is to devalue it and to demean it.

Because this condition is a bittersweet privilege, a paradox of insight and madness; because it breaks your heart wide open and cuts you to the quick, yet there is honey on the razor's edge. Because this condition is often portrayed as simply one of emotional highs and lows, but there is far more to it: it alters how one hears music, sees art and reads poetry, and I want to explore the psyche's accents and alterations.

Because manic depression seems to me a misunderstood condition, and I want to describe it for those who have never experienced it but who perhaps know someone with it. Inevitably, I must portray my own experience, but it is an illness with considerable commonality and I want to describe my journey through it for those who have experienced their own journeys, because what is individual can speak to the general, and if this book can befriend just one person in that terrifying loneliness, it will be worth writing.

Because, at the heart of it all, I lost my words and found them again with a gratitude and a devotion which any writer living in service to their art may understand. Language and literature are the longest loves of my life and in their signs I saw my way. If this book leans on them – on etymology, on poetry and on precise and precious words, it is because I know nothing wiser, I love nothing so much and I trust nothing more than the truths of language, the greatest artwork ever made, created over thousands of years with the signatures of millions.

How to describe this crazed state? What are the words which capture manic depression, in particular in its mixed-state form? What are the terms through which one feels understood and by means of which other people could understand? 'Tristimania' – coined by eighteenth-century American psychiatrist Benjamin Rush – tells it true to me. Rush may have meant it as a precise shading of melancholia, but it works perfectly for the *tristesse*, the distress coupled with mania, which a mixed-state bipolar episode provokes.

The Old English term *wōd*, meaning 'mad' or 'frenzied', was replaced by the word 'mad' in Middle English. 'Mad' denotes the crazy state, but it connotes little. *Wōd*, though, carries connotations and etymological links which give insight of a whole other order into the madness of manic depression. The Indo-European root is *wet* – to blow, inspire and spiritually arouse. *Wet* is the source of the Latin *vates*, meaning 'seer' or 'poet', and also source of the Old Irish

word *faith*, meaning 'poet'. *Wōd* is linked to Old English *woþ*, meaning 'sound', 'melody', 'song', and cognate with Old Norse *óðr*,
meaning 'mad, frantic, furious, violent'. (As a noun, *óðr* means
'mind, wit, soul, sense' and 'song, poetry'.) *Wōd* is linked to Odin,
too, god of war and wisdom, shamanism and poetry. The Roman
historian Tacitus considered that Mercury was the chief god of the
Germanic tribes, almost certainly because he saw in Odin the qualities of Mercury. Odin, like Mercury, was a 'guide of souls' and was
said to have brought poetry to humankind. *Wōd* also gives us
Wōdensday, Wednesday, the day of Mercury, and – appropriately –
this was the day of the week when I had been at my most *wōd*.

Some people find manic-depressive breakdown a form of spiritual experience, offering a sense of divine insight. Many people with
manic depression create (or need) music and poetry. With the word
wōd, everything links and the savage beauties of this madness
become more eloquent. Looked at one way, it is medical. Looked
at another, it is spiritual. Looked at a third way, it is poetry. Or,
indeed, love.

In medical terms, like most people with manic depression, most
of the time I have no symptoms. Also, like many people with it, I
can see a genetic pattern. An episode of manic depression can be
seen to have a medical or psychological aetiology including being
affected by lack of sleep, stress, alcohol and psychological trauma
(particularly involving humiliation), or loss. Psychologist Richard P.
Bentall writes of studies which show that there is a high rate of
'intrusive' events in the weeks preceding psychosis, including
unwanted sexual propositions. People with manic depression also
have an increased sensitivity to light and, according to Bentall, sleep
deprivation may provoke mania; he also notes that before the advent
of modern lighting, when people were more accustomed to longer

nocturnal darknesses, the full moon would have had more of an effect on insomnia, and there would surely have been a greater link between the lunar and the lunatic.

Lovesickness was once considered to be a medical illness. Its symptoms included loss of appetite, headache, fever, palpitations and insomnia. Some medieval writings describe lovesickness in terms of symptoms which today would be seen as those of bipolar disorder: so a person diagnosed as lovesick may display rapid mood swings from manic laughter to the anguished weeping of depression.

The electricity of mania coursing through you does predispose you to fall in love and, yes, in the months of recovery, I did 'fall' in love. Or, rather, slip up on a banana skin; daftly, inadvertently, unrequitably, mistakenly, serio-comically, as the guy in question was completely off limits.

This particular unrequitable love wasn't in the slightest bit sad. I didn't mind. In fact, I quite liked it, because it was one of the ultimately safe love affairs, like my other grand passions for Rupert Brooke, Michel de Montaigne, Dafydd ap Gwilym and (life-long) Shakespeare. The thing about love is this: I love being in love. I love loving people and animals, words, flowers and jokes. I love the way love courses through the spirit, how it brightens everything around you, how it inspirits you, lifts the drooping head of aquilegia, raises the downcast expression, brings more colours to the rainbow. This is what manic depression does, too. In the throes of it, I feel an incandescent sensitivity by which everything is only too much alive and calling. My nerves are exposed: the world is ferociously present. In love with mania as I was, falling in love with a person was something of a misattribution.

Various anthropologists have argued that, although our society interprets certain psychological conditions as a medical issue, other cultures have construed exactly the same states of mind as shamanic, divinely inspired wisdom, and those possessed of such insight may be honoured. Professor of psychiatry Richard Warner, noting the work of Mircea Eliade and Black Elk, describes how 'In non-industrial cultures throughout the world, the hallucinations and altered states of consciousness produced by psychosis, fasting, sleep deprivation, social isolation and contemplation and hallucinogenic drug use are often a prerequisite for gaining shamanic power.' As Mircea Eliade writes, mental illness reveals a shamanic vocation, and shamanic initiation is equivalent to the cure: 'The famous Yakut shaman Tüspüt (that is, "fallen from the sky") had been ill at the age of twenty; he began to sing, and felt better . . . he needed to shamanize; if he went for a long time without doing so, he did not feel well.' (An Icarus, by any other name, would fly as high and fall as steeply.)

Dr Orhan Öztürk, a Turkish psychiatrist, writes: 'A person may be hallucinated or delusional, but as long as he is not destructive or very unstable he may not be considered insane . . . Such a person may sometimes be considered to have a supernatural capacity for communication with the spirit world and may therefore be regarded with reverence and awe.'

The medieval historian Giraldus Cambrensis (Gerald of Wales) describes a phenomenon which would most likely be understood as mental illness today but which in his own time was taken as prophecy:

> Among the Welsh there are certain individuals called Awenyddion who behave as if they are possessed . . . When you consult them about some problem, they immediately go into a trance and lose control of their senses . . . if you listen carefully to what they say

you will receive the solution to your problem . . . They seem to receive this gift of divination through visions which they see in their dreams. Some of them have the impression that honey or sugary milk is being smeared on their mouths; others say that a sheet of paper with words written on it is pressed against their lips.

American anthropologist Ruth Benedict describes how Siberian shamans 'are individuals who by submission to the will of the spirits have been cured of a grievous illness . . . Some, during the period of the call, are violently insane for several years; others irresponsible to the point where they have to be constantly watched lest they wander off in the snow and freeze to death . . . It is the shamanistic practice which constitutes their cure.'

In the time of Plato and Socrates, the gods were thought to communicate with poets and priests through inspired madness and *enthusiasm*; the passion of the god within, *en-theos*. 'Madness comes from God, whereas sober sense is merely human,' according to Socrates, in *Phaedrus*: far from being stigmatizing, 'Madness, provided it comes as the gift of heaven, is the channel by which we receive the greatest blessings.' Dionysus, meanwhile, subject to great agony and equally great ecstasy, is the god in the grip of this wildness. Robert Burton, author of *The Anatomy of Melancholy*, wrote of Aristotle's view that melancholia caused men to experience 'many times a divine ravishment, and a kind of *enthusiasmus* . . . which stirreth them up to be excellent Philosophers, Poets, Prophets, etc.'

In *Ion*, Plato has Socrates say: 'For the poet is a light and winged and holy thing, and there is no invention in him until he has been inspired and is out of his senses, and the mind is no longer in him . . . for not by art does the poet sing, but by power divine.' Oscar Wilde referred to 'the old fancy which made the poet's art an enthusiasm, a form of divine possession'.

For the early Church Fathers, David was the greatest of all poets, able to move between divine gift and human consciousness. Historical figures such as the medieval Margery Kempe – who would today be considered psychotic – were considered mystics. If you see visions, are you delusional and sick, or a spiritual visionary? Ancient Norse bards considered poetry to be a gift of the gods which was then shaped by human skill. Traditional Arabian belief in djinns suggested a sense of being possessed by spirits who gave people knowledge but could also drive them mad.

Alexandre Dumas wrote of the poet Gérard de Nerval's episodes of madness: 'Our poor Gérard, for the men of science he is a sick man and needs treatment, while for us he is simply more the story-teller, more the dreamer, more spiritual, more happy or more sad than ever.' The link between manic depression and the artistic temperament has been much studied, including by Kay Redfield Jamison in her fascinating book *Touched with Fire*, which, like all her work, is priceless in the way it comprehends, counsels and consoles the manic-depressive psyche.

Interestingly, one feature of hypomania and mania is hyperacusis – an increased awareness of objects in one's environment – which is certainly an aspect of artistic sensitivity. In general, manic depression is a condition of passion, the ability to feel pain, to create and to love. The word 'passion', in its root, means 'to suffer' (as in 'the Passion of Christ'). Olive trees were, for Vincent van Gogh, associated with Christ's Passion, and, if I look at his painting *Les Oliviers* (*Olive Trees*), painted while he was in the asylum at Saint-Rémy, I see it instantly: the suffering art in his agitated, manic swirls, the turbulence which cannot be calmed. In this Passion, the trees are screaming. No wonder he sliced off his own ear, for the world was shrieking at him and his psyche could not be quieted.

An Anglican clergyman of the seventeenth century specialized in treating people he called 'unquiet of mind' (the beautiful phrase adapted for the title of Kay Redfield Jamison's record of her own illness), and it is a deft definition, a listening definition, for those in manic-depressive crisis do hear the sounds of madness within, the weird singing of a high-tension wire or a wind-wolf and, indeed, hear the sudden silence as mind crashes inward during a conversation.

People in mania often don't write about it, say psychologists, and cannot remember it until they are in that state again. Richard Bentall comments on the 'poor descriptions offered in the classic literature of psychiatry' and suggests that 'likely there is something about the manic state that makes it almost impossible to portray in words . . . accounts seem curiously incomplete. It is as if the break from normal functioning during an episode is so severe that the mind, on returning to sanity, cannot comprehend it.'

I'm not surprised. When your mind is in flight you don't leave tracks on the ground, so there are no prints, neither footprints nor printed letters on the page. But I felt fiercely that I had to take notes during this *wōdness*, that I had to mark the tracks of its passage. I've trained myself to jot down notes wherever I am: in the dark, while walking, while driving, while climbing, half asleep, underwater, in deserts and icescapes. This was just another form of difficult terrain, and I leant on my habit and training.

In my previous episode, years before, I had taken no notes, and had had no comprehension of what was happening; instead, I had to rely on the observation of others. My flatmate at the time said she felt she was helplessly watching me float upwards, borne skywards, holding the string of a helium balloon, rising, dangerously rising. She wanted to grab me and pull me down, but I slipped ever upwards, out of sight. The painter Benjamin Haydon, a friend of John Keats, used a similar image: 'I have been like a man with air balloons under his armpits and ether in his soul.'

Describing mania is like a sundial trying to tether the shadow of a sun gone AWOL, zigzagging across the sky. Sometimes I felt weirdly still, both weightless and vigilant, hyper-aware like an inconcrete meerkat fascinated by a mirage. Sometimes, the opposite of wistful, I felt wist*less*, recklessly so. Sometimes my mind was a giddy, vertiginous mosaic of turquoise lettered in gold. Sometimes the restless energy coursing through me was like being possessed by a divinity lightfoot in pursuit of feathers: shimmering, galloping and surging.

Rilke described his breakdown as a 'boundless storm, a hurricane of the spirit', and manic-depressive people often use images of the natural world. Shelley described Byron as 'mad as the winds', and it was an image Byron echoed: 'If I must sail let it be on the ocean no matter how stormy'; and he writes of the voyagings of poetry, of sailing 'in the wind's eye' and bringing back images to 'counterbalance human woes'.

But the flight cannot last. When mania falls to depression, it is as if the storm clouds have congealed, solidified to dank fat. Time itself goes stale. Depression, swollen and greedy, is a slug-glutton, feeding on the tender green soul.

It is payback time.

Sometimes the payback is literal, as people have spent and squandered money, giving it away and racking up debts. When mania turns to depression, the payback is also emotional – a sense of guilt about what sufferers have done, and taxingly difficult repayment, the Danegeld of guilty gold, particularly when manic depression has encouraged overspending oneself sexually in impetuous affairs. Darian Leader points out that the Greek word *mania*, usually translated as 'madness' or 'frenzy', in its plural form evoked the Eumenides, 'whose function it was to pursue those who had not, precisely, paid their dues'.

Manic depression can't balance the books, and it struggles in a mercurial seesaw of credit and debt, extravagance and penitence, exuberance and recoil, the endlessly kinetic commerce of Mercury.

Manic depression is more usually called by the chilly term 'bipolar', a bipedal term; mathematical, binary and wrong. 'Mania' leans to the waltz, falling and rising in threes.

In mania, the mind dances faster than usual: thoughts are quicker and speech is quicker. It also feels like an increase of 'quickness' – of aliveness or vitality – which is paid for in depression later at the price of an increase of deadness. ('I felt a Funeral, in my brain,' as Emily Dickinson wrote.)

The kinetic quality of mania involves many moving parts: physical energy in the need to keep moving, to run, to spend energy of all kinds. Money moves quickly in mania's hands; it runs, its currency (from *correre* in Latin, 'to run') is spent at speed.

People's speech runs fast in mania. Coleridge's intense talkativeness 'dazzled bystanders by containing too many ideas in too few words', according to his biographer Richard Holmes. Sometimes the speed of connection in one's thoughts is so fast that the steps are invisible and a lackbrain hearer may dismiss it as disconnected, whereas it is the result of an over-connected mind, going at the speed of light, faster than the speed of sound.

Welcome to the foundry.

Here we have Mercury or Hermes' half-brother Hephaestus, the blacksmith of genius. And here we have melting of bells. Hear the silent temples. You may steeple your fingers at your head and pray, aspire to the pealing of gold, but madness has your feet to the flames, molten and made into bullets you can shoot – straight through your temples.

Mixed-state manic depression is manic depression on speed. In mixed state, one's moods oscillate within hours, even minutes; a flux of unplannable ecstasy and unpredictable agony.

The hurricanes within want serenity but get doldrums. The doldrums want breeze but get hurricanes.

As this episode for me began, appropriately, in the autumn or fall of the year with a literal fall down a rabbit hole, it was a falling into madness of a paradoxical sort; a soaring fall, a falling flight, tripping the switches. ('I feel like I'm tripping,' I said often to friends at the high points.) It was a sick, lurching helter-skelter of the psyche. The fall from hypomania to depression may be a matter of quicksilver timing, but then mania re-erupts through depression's stupor.

It is self-provoking, this gyre, self-swerving around an elastic axis, turning and turning. The licked finger circles and circles the rim of the glass till a wail rises and the glass shatters itself, shards of broken-heartedness which will stab the barefoot psyche.

I developed an obsessive terror of losing things, particularly my notebooks, which I clutched at compulsively, sometimes every minute, checking they were still there. If I left my house, I often had to walk with my hand in my satchel, fingers touching the pages. I had to check every packet of empty Rizla papers several times before I burnt it, in case I'd written a thought on one of them and would lose it. Scraps of paper, shopping lists, odd reminders, the little docket with the next doctor's appointment written on it; all were nervously guarded. I felt real panic when I thought I'd lost a hat, and emailed and phoned friends trying to find it. Mad as a hatter, Mercury brimming. If I can't even hold on to a notebook, how can I hold on to my sanity? was my reasoning. If I lose my hat it shows that I am losing my mind: lostness was the pivot of my panic.

And then I crashed my computer, losing at a stroke the ability to receive the slips of sanity my geographically removed friends were sending me. It happened late one night. I was drunk. Both my common sense and my computer were running dangerously low on battery power. A red warning sign popped up on the screen telling me to turn the computer off immediately or there'd be trouble. It was an odd but precise parallel to what had already happened to me the day I went mad: I ignored the red warning sign, and then on the sudden the screen froze. True to its word, my computer wheeped and fizzled out to black. It never worked again. The motherboard was fucked. I knew the feeling.

I could borrow a friend's computer, from time to time, but I hated not being able to read and re-read my friends' sane, kind, helpful messages at any time. The loss of that easy access made me even more isolated. At this point, too, it was becoming clear that it wasn't safe for me to drive. I didn't care much about an accident involving only myself, but I was concerned about a passenger of mine or anyone else on the roads.

Everything seemed to be metaphor. Car crash for breakdown. Motherboard for rationality. Notebook for mind. Hat for head. But, in a more extensive way, metaphor was becoming more true, if not more actual, than reality. Metaphor had more significance. There was meaning in this madness which I must find, I thought. Metaphor matters in madness. Matters so much that you could say metaphor is the material of madness, the mothering tongue of the madstruck mind, *mater* of it all. I could feel the metaphoric weight of things in my mind, heavy as a mountain. More importantly, metaphors alone could bear the weight which my mind, heavy with intensity, placed on them. Metaphor was strong enough. Reality wasn't. Reality weighed so lightly on me that the actuality of the entire Cambrian mountain range was a skittering colt in frantic canter. Significance shifted. Gravity, heft and import were all located in the metaphorical world.

I was dwelling in the realms of metaphor. At the beginning of this madness, my main metaphor was ocean, being at the shoreline before the tsunami; later, I felt like a broken boat in sea surges of storm, in waves that would wreck me. Over and over again, I felt I was drowning. In a brief and brilliant moment, my realm was starlight; I felt I was flying in the flickering world of utter space. For months, though, my realm was mountains. The edge. The abyss. The death zone at the peak.

What does it mean, to live in metaphors? I was perfectly aware that my actual physical self was sitting next to my woodstove, or in the garden shed, or at the piano; I knew this was the literal and tangible truth, but this was not the whole truth. The wider, deeper truth could only be told in metaphor. 'Meta-phor', in its etymology, means a carrying-across of attributes from one thing to another. Metaphor also carries meaning across from one person to another; it is a messenger bearing messages. The god of metaphor is Mercury; this is the realm of the Trickster, carrying things across borders, living in the in-between.

If a person uses a metaphor, they are carrying themselves over, towards the listener, but in madness this need becomes infinitely more intense. In a manic-depressive episode, metaphors are heavy with meaning, and the metaphors one chooses must carry an almost unbearable weight. This, I think, is why people are so stubborn about repeating the precise metaphors which tell their truth. Gérard de Nerval saw depression as a black sun. Poet Les Murray, Winston Churchill and others describe it as the 'black dog'. Some say they are in an 'abyss' or a 'black hole'; others that they are 'drowning'. For the person in crisis, these images are carrying a burden of significance which listeners, be they doctors, psychiatrists or friends, need to appreciate.

When a person is ill, a metaphor is not a decoration, not a trivial curlicue of Eng. Lit., not a doily on the conversational table; rather, it is a desperate attempt to send out an SOS, to give the listener their coordinates, because they are losing themselves. *I am on Cader Idris, just before the first peak after the path leaves the lake: do you read me? Over.* The perilous geography where my psyche was situated. Situated but dis-located, alone and pathless. I had to be meticulously precise in giving the latitude of my madness, the longitude of my scraps of insight. I was lost and urgently needed to be found, to be located by someone who could (as shamans say) send their souls out to find mine. In terms of our culture, one way of doing this is surprisingly simple: listeners need to hear the metaphors and stay with them. My doctor used my metaphors with almost unfaltering precision, and I felt safer for it. In all the hours of appointments, there was only one time I remember when he used a completely different metaphor to the one I'd just used, and I couldn't say anything. It was a broken moment, and I was lost, all over again. But every other time, by using my metaphors, he made me feel located, as if I could hold his hand and follow the way he knew and I'd forgotten, back to safety.

In *Don Quixote*, the delusional Quixote is treated by the doctor

(Cervantes himself), who aims to cure his madness by working within his lunacy, curing him through the very terms he uses. It is crucial that listeners do not scramble the message or scumble the precision of the image. If the listener can stay within the terrain of the exact metaphor the speaker is using, they will feel more findable, more reachable. (*I read you. What's the mountain weather report? Stay away from the cliff edges* . . .) But if, by contrast, the reply confuses the image (*I understand. You're feeling very low. You're in a dark pit*), then the person in crisis will feel more lost, more isolated and more endangered.

People in psychiatric crisis are living more in their minds than in the actual world, and words have an extraordinary power. They can swap places with things; they can crush, poison and kill. They can also give life, illuminate and heal. *Logos* is indeed a divine principle: words create reality.

My need for metaphor was ferocious: I clung to it as if my life depended on it, as if my SOS from Cader were a text message tapped out on a dying phone with low charge and a weak signal sent to the Mountain Rescue Service. Help. I am mad. North-north-west. Eleven o'clock on the dial, moving dangerously into the midnight hour.

Sometimes, though, I had a positive sense of the metaphoric terrain; I was in another land, the other world. In a compliment to our species, I'd suggest humanity cannot bear too much *mere* reality, deadened reality unenlivened by significance, meaning, poetry or art. I wanted to escape the tethers of dogmatic rationalism, to say that this way of seeing is not enough, the mind needs more. It is a yearning for the ultimate, for God, for the divine, for art, for poetry, and I found myself longing to dwell elsewhere, where the mind can dream, awake. A yearning not to climb an actual mountain but rather the mountain's reflection in still lakes.

Madness is a way of seeing aligned to the shadow rather than the object which casts it. Madness is a way of hearing attuned to the echo rather than the melody which causes it. The other world. The uncertain world. The peripheral vision. The idea-world, where metaphor is like the 'sympathetic string' on an instrument, which is usually unplayed but resounds in sympathetic resonance to the playing of the main string, most strongly at either the same tone or an octave interval. The main string actually played is not as important as the sympathetic string which sings its negative capability in a resonance of gold. Matter doesn't matter as much as the immaterial world. Metaphor is not of matter and yet how much it matters.

The literal world has a metaphoric penumbra of significance, and this is where the world glows, the halo of events; for nothing is only real. It is real and it is ideal, as if the psyche's metaphoric idea of something is always the augmented version, the Greater: as if Idea in the human mind has grandeur far beyond Reality and Plato was right all along. It is the mindset of fairy tales, where every encounter has enormity and significance, where people are hugely good or hugely destructive. There are trolls, kind kings, good animal companions.

People in a crisis of manic depression are said to be prone to idealizing people or demonizing them, though probably a better way of phrasing it is 'to demonize' and 'to angelize'. I certainly did that medically, angelizing my doctor and demonizing the psychiatrist, and many memoirs seem to do the same. Both extremes are Ideal, from the realm of Idea. Metaphoric angels. Metaphoric demons.

Because just as the mind makes distinctions between actual mountain and metaphoric Mountain, so it creates distinctions between the actual, sweet-hearted friend and the metaphoric Angel, between the actual, highly skilled doctor and the metaphoric Saviour. As if the metaphorical vision capitalized the heart of things. As if it crushed everything to its quintessence, the fifth quality, the purest ethereal nature of things, as if I saw the Ocean of the ocean, the Moon of the moon, the Candle of the candle, the Solstice of the solstice, the Midnight of midnight with the I of my i. Alone.

But living in the world of metaphor can exact a high price. I was very lonely. There is an enormous difference between loneliness, isolation and solitude. Solitude has a sweet serenity, frictionless as flame licking itself. Loneliness is where solitude becomes too poignant and the flame begins to burn you. Isolation, though, has a punitive edge; illness can isolate you and so can the simple fact of my profession; the loneliness of the long-distance writer. Mostly, I love solitude all day and company all night, but I became violently lonely in this illness, not because I lacked company but because I became fussy as a cat over who I could be with, and when.

I spent most of my time alone in depression's one-person tragedy, feeling as if I were both the chorus, reading ahead in the script, and also the isolate agonist in a killing tale. I imprisoned myself behind walls of silence: the unanswered telephone ringing itself into oblivion; the kind-hearted emails, not ignored exactly but certainly unanswered.

Alone, swollen with self-loathing, self-revolted, I saw myself once like a rotting octopus, tentacles of dying flesh suffocating me, poison seeping colourlessly through my veins, all my pointless life in cancelled colours draining into abnegation, the nearly nothing meaninglessness of obliteration.

Privacy can be dangerous, because it gives someone in crisis a place to hide their intentions, to conceal many things, chief among them suicidality. As Kay Redfield Jamison comments: 'The privacy of the mind is an impermeable barrier.'

I craved solitude but I also craved company to ward off the devastations of my loneliness. The difficulty was that each need collided with its opposite so that when I was alone I could become desperate to be in company but as soon as I was with people I would often need to be alone. At worst, I'd withdraw instantly as if snatching my hand back from nettles.

I felt an urgent need to be understood and to be among people with whom I could be unlonely, so that I would not be trapped in solitude but could be released into telling talk. Sometimes I was alone, wanting company but unable to do the one necessary thing: I wished someone would just walk straight into my house, find me wherever I was – in bed, in the corner of the garden, by the stove – and hold my head, find the gentling words; the psyche-whisperers who could find the way towards me, letting words of light, of truth, of love, spool out into the air.

I yearned for people with minds of silk – delicate-thoughted, smooth against my sore, bruised psyche, soft as mare's tail cloud and yet with the tensile strength of spidersilk, five times stronger than steel, strong enough to withstand being near madness but subtle enough, sweet enough, silken enough, for me to be able to touch it. Maybe I could use that silk as a lifeline, could hold it to cross back over into the healthy world, finding the silk road between continents of minds.

But, alone, that transaction of sensitivity, that commerce of silk, sometimes seemed impossible, the risks too great. What if I couldn't speak? What if they tried to reach me and couldn't? My disappointment: their hurt. Depressed people can make those around them feel badly rejected, and my sadness and madness could (and did) ripple out beyond me, my rejections causing further hurt to other people. It still pains me that many people around me were hurt by my inability to reach out to them and ask for help, because when I closed down I held on to just a tiny number of close old friends.

As far as the larger world was concerned, I tried to Act Normal. Being mad is, to put it bluntly, embarrassing. In manic depression, it is too easy to lose one's inhibitions, and the ordinary traffic of the world is weirdly dissonant: codes of behaviour and decorum seem peculiarly frivolous compared to the fury of emotions within.

Sometimes the incongruous disjunction of the private and public worlds is as ludicrous as it is heartbreaking. The poet William Cowper's *Memoir* records his breakdown in 1763, triggered by undertaking a job of a very public nature, as Clerk of the Journals in the House of Lords, and finding his suitability for the job questioned. High-stress work in the public eye was the opposite of what he really needed, which was a vast and protected privacy. As he became more ill, the breakthroughs from the public world into his private soul seemed maddening interruptions. In particular, his laundress and her husband always seemed to be busy too near him in his chambers, and at one point, suicidal, he tried to hang himself in his bedroom while the laundress was in the dining room: she 'must have passed by the bedchamber door . . . while I was hanging upon it'.

Depressed and vulnerable, I was frightened of clumsiness. Stupidity felt as brutal and painful as being punched. I felt as if I were walking in crystal forests with stained-glass skies and crassness was as violent as swinging concrete arms; words like dumb-bells; cranes for eyes. At times, even good-natured bonhomie seemed a terrible cacophony of raw trumpets baying, with violins used as percussion for gross toasts, a piano lid a drinks table, clarinets stuck, reeds down, into the ground, used as flagpoles for Ingerland bunting, and flutes stolen as sticks to crack heads open.

Most of the time, like a sick cat, I wanted to hide unseen in a dark corner, trembling with the toxicity of madness streaming through my veins. I couldn't stand being mothered, but I sought consolation. I craved understanding, but I staggered inwardly at the ways in which manic depression could be grossly misunderstood. One friend's brother, heavily into diet-related health, offered his opinion: 'You eat too much wheat.' I felt winded by the abyss between my experience and his comprehension, as if he really thought that toast and marmalade could convulse the mind to psychosis, as if too many cheese sandwiches could cause suicidal ideation.

From time to time, I sought out particular friends for particular reasons: one, because he was authoritative by nature, and he was willing and able to outshout the siren voices in my head; another, because she could join me wherever I was: if I was kite-high with a mile-long streamer of giggles bubbling behind me, she could find me there and laugh with me, but when I sank and my heart had plunged like a broken kite to the Earth, suddenly, she was there, too, right beside me, serious, kind and quiet.

My friends were all different, but the nature of their friendship was alike. They were constant, loyal and enduring. I am still appalled at the time-consuming nature of an illness like this, and I am beyond gratitude for their generosity; they gave and gave and gave without end and without knowing how long it would last. I could count on them, knowing that they would hold themselves strong. If they had not seemed strong, I couldn't have leant on them, and it wasn't that they didn't have their own difficulties and sadnesses in that long year but rather that they took immense care to hold firm in the hours they spent with me and to be weak, if they needed to be, elsewhere.

One gave me a bird's nest, woven with the softest feathers and moss, with a note tucked inside saying 'A nest for your spirit'. One, on a horribly bleak morning in winter-spring, left a tray of gorgeous pansies on my doorstep. One, who lives too far away for me to see her easily, called me often on the phone. She could hear the silent words between my breaths and gauge how low I was by all I could not say. They protected me, standing between me and the world, gentle sides towards me and tough sides outward, and they were fierce to ward away from me anything or anyone who was unhelpful. I was sheltered by their shields – an unassailable, interlocked circle.

My cats were also acutely important when I was ill. The poet Christopher Smart, who was manic depressive, spent seven years in a mental asylum. He was allowed to keep a cat, and wrote the loveliest ode ever dedicated to a cat, writing of his cat, Jeoffry:

> *For there is nothing sweeter than his peace when at rest.*
> *For there is nothing brisker than his life when in motion.*

Now, as I write, my cat Tom is asleep on my study floor. He is using two of my small black notebooks from that year of illness as a pillow for his head. He is a feral cat but has been with me since kittenhood and is more attached to me than any cat I've known. What do they do, these pets, for our savaged psyches? They are company; they breathe near us, and that in itself is consolation. They are more than happy to wake in the middle of the night and pad downstairs to sit with us in the kitchen. 'For he keeps the Lord's watch in the night against the adversary,' wrote Smart. They need us to feed them and, at my worst, this responsibility was more pressing than the need to feed myself but knowing that I could at least perform this task was helpful. They offer affection without analysis. They are an exercise in instant mindfulness: wholly purring, wholly stretching, wholly sunbasking, wholly catnip-toy-mouse-chasing. They cannot but live in an eternal present and do so beguilingly, drawing us, too, towards the glow at the heart of now.

Though my sleep was short, the medication made me sleep furiously – that phrase which Gideon Koppel used to title his exquisite film, precisely because Chomsky had said it had no meaning. If I slept furiously, I also felt a life force furious within, of green life in a green flame flowing, and it seemed both to conjure and confound the suicidal thoughts which devilled me. Mania was like a Faust in my mind, paradoxically both calling up the demon suicide and at the same time driving it off in rage: when suicide seemed to tinge the edge of my vision, mania roared at it: *Stand Where I Can See You. And FUCK OFF.*

Maybe the sleep of depression protects you, through its anaesthesia, from something worse, from the pain that would drive you to suicide. Perhaps, further, that's part of the reason why mixed-state hypomania is so dangerous; because its depressions are sleepless, and that sleeplessness feeds on itself, self-cannibalizing. In sleepless mania, the mind is yellow-dizzy with a turbulence of colour, the air licks it with tongues of fire, flowers bow their petals like violinists and are bent to the applause of a rapturous wind while even the shadows of things are brilliant and burning. (Van Gogh knew.)

The ferocity of life sought the idea of death like an artist might: a painter demanding chiaroscuro – dark light shining. Vitality connected me with every living thing and filled me with an acute love for the world's life forms, for every bird, every tree, every mountain. Nothing seemed to have its normal surface; everything and everyone seemed semi-permeable. This, too, is the over-connected aspect of mania, and one of its most profound experiences is the feeling of being able to step over the threshold of 'Other' without quibbling about species difference, or language, or the expectation of either boundary-mind or barrier-body. This contains the blunt psychiatric concept of the manic 'disinhibition' but goes far beyond its crude enactions (taking one's clothes off in public; being wholly inappropriate) into the precious experience of finding oneself porous to the world. It can thus be a spiritual experience and an artistic one. Keats's famous 'negative capability' comes close to explaining this feeling that the psyche's skin is transparent, and the psyche of others can seem so. It is a glorious trespass, weirdly observant, and often correctly intuitive, steeped in deep empathy, a fellow-feeling. Empathy, incidentally, is one of the key markers of manic depression identified by Darian Leader. No wonder so many people feeling manic and hypomanic want to have sex with loads of people, but that is so literal and therefore not as interesting as this extensive, metaphysical love, not crudely 'making love' but rather noticing the love surrounding every human, every animal, the transcendent betweenness.

A friend was ill, with a breast cancer scare, and wanted me with her for some of the treatment, and we choreographed a dance of mutual care. I went to see her in London. But on the train I found myself desperately trying not to scream. I wanted to get off the train and do – what, exactly? Bizarrely, of all things, I wanted to find a policeman and ask for help. As if I needed someone else's power, and my mind suddenly read 'power' literally. I had no idea what I would have asked them to do – call a doctor? Take me home? Hold my hand? Tell me a joke? What? I do not know. All of the above would have been helpful, but I was scared of their reaction. Transport police are in fact accustomed to coping with people who are experiencing psychiatric problems, and are trained to deal with them. *Sorry, Officer, it's a bit of an emergency . . . I need you to tell me a good joke.* Yes, I know how absurd that sounds, but it felt as if a joke could create a sane link between my mind and someone else's more quickly than anything else.

Once I'd got to London, I had a soaring moment when I wanted to take my shoes off and run across the city, barefoot and naked, as if by doing so I could join myself to the roaring and jubilant pandemonium of cityness. My voice of reason stepped in firmly, quoting that familiar line: 'The thing about inviting trouble is that trouble usually accepts.' But I wanted to hold on to the spirit of that wish, the racing of naked flame without the embarrassment (and dangerous stupidity) of its actualization. On a bus going to my friend's house, I watched a father with his three young children, and I felt a wave of utter love for them all, creatures as we all are of fire and love and need and hope. This sensual fire connects – one's ardour easily sets another's alight – but I wanted to let it run to the ethereal rather than the corporeal until I could cry out to the sky itself that I loved it.

I was with my friend at a hospital appointment post-surgery. I was meant to be there as her Sensible Friend. (Ahem.) Trying with all my might to stay engaged, I managed to jot down the right questions we needed to ask and even get the answers. We came to the crucial appointment when she was told she was in the clear. She went into a shocked state of vertiginous relief. In the moment of delight and love, I slipped on a mental banana skin and fell into cartoon: Desperate Dan unleashed in Vizland. Hullabaloo – like a rubber boomerang made of chewing gum and powered by farts – exploded in my mind, and I started giggling terribly. One of the nurses was looking at me uneasily. 'I'm so sorry,' I gasped, 'my friend's just had breast cancer and I'm hypomanic, so we're both off our tits.'

Then my friend lost her umbrella and I lost her. It only lasted a few minutes, but it was as disturbing as a dream where everything is almost exactly as you know it to be, but with the crucial bit (my friend) entirely missing. When we found each other, we went out for lunch to celebrate her results and, although she was pleased, she was still weak and shaky. And there, as she sat opposite me, I could see her wings. Black and shining, her wingtips were tilted to hope, curious for sky, quizzically trying for a fledgling happiness. It was so right for her situation after the flightless and frightening cancer weeks, and I told her what I could see. Once again, I didn't think they really existed, but it was like seeing an actualized metaphor, and I sketched her, and both of us hummed the Beatles' 'Blackbird singing'.

The Christmas lights along Regent Street were like reindeer horns and made me feel trippy, the shoots and offshoots and offshoots of the offshoots, all curling and dendritic, like a visible and outward design of invisible and inward mind-lines, how one thought shoots off to another and another. My mind lit up and my heart felt full of love for my friend, and we passed a shop selling mugs and bought one for her saying 'JOY'.

It is ravenous, this hypomanic state; all-consuming and auto-consuming, and I could feel it yearning towards mania, wanting a higher reach. But aces in this bipolar game are both high and low, and after eventually managing to sleep that night, I woke with my face in spasm, muscles leaping through reflex of emotions unbidden. In this crash, London was a terrifying place to be, and

I wondered how I could manage to get home. I needed to be near my doctor.

Technically, he was a GP, but more truly he was a mind doctor, a psyche-*iatros*, as the root of the word 'psychiatrist' attests, the most gifted doctor I'd ever met. He was also, in the deepest sense of the word, a healer. I had told him that in one early appointment, and he had gently turned the compliment aside, in a self-deprecating *only-doing-my-job* kind of gesture.

I held on to these appointments as if my life depended on them, and this is no exaggeration. I felt at the time, and still feel now, that my doctor saved my life. In the course of the crisis, which lasted into weeks and months, I saw him dozens of times and, partway through, I began to wonder what it felt like to listen to a mad person so desperate to talk, so much and so often. Madness forces you to concentrate on it. It is attention-seeking because it wants an audience. Madness wants to paint its vision so the world can see what the human mind is capable of seeing. It wants to play its passions so the world can hear the song. It wants to write and speak because it seeks to be understood and to understand itself. It wants to utter – to outer – its inner knowledge. It is as if the human mind, on its continuum from normal middle C to the upper reaches and lower depths, needs some people to play the highest Cs and to be played by the cavernous bass, so that everyone may know of those realms, even if they themselves are never dwellers there.

It is troubling to find oneself in mid-flight and uninterruptable, hijacking people's attention. I suddenly remembered that joke about the egotist at a party: *Is it solipsistic in here, or is it just me?*; and told my doctor, who laughed. After that, I tried to save up any joke I heard or remembered, and take it to appointments to lighten his load of listening.

I feel sorry for doctors: we take our dodgy psyches, our warts and bad breath, our boring aches and nondescript pains, our malfunctions and mishumours and moods, our putrid life experiences and biliousness and vaginal discharges and itchy foreskins and diarrhoea, and our bums-with-grapes and our leaking noses and eyes, and our swellings and protuberances and our history-ofs and our tears and our sleeplessness, and our skinninesses and our obesities and our corns and earwax and ingrowths and outgrowths and groins and acne: and we stick it all in front of the doctor, all this dirt and ugliness. Good doctors leave me in awe.

Several people – particularly those in the caring professions – have asked me what exactly my doctor did that was so helpful. It seems important, particularly because so many people in manic-depressive crisis feel acutely aware of what goes wrong with their medical care. So: what did he do right?

He listened, deeply. I felt as if he let my words into his mind, so that he could re-hear my words right inside himself and re-listen if necessary. There was a musicality to his empathy. He heard in resonances, making of himself the sympathetic string. I felt utterly – unbelievably – understood. Because he listened to my metaphors, I felt he was willing to walk with me in the landscapes of my mind. When I was stranded up a mountain, the one thing that kept me safe was a slender but strong rope which he held, and I trusted him not to let it go. It seems significant that many people in manic-depressive crisis, including me, speak of ropes, lifelines, threads and linking things, because this madness is sharply focused on connection and disconnection, from the neural pathways of the mind to the Trickster paths and the relational pathways between people. In the weirdscape I walked in, he was my lead climber, guiding in line with the etymological heart of doctoring. He told me the etymology of 'doctor', from *docere*: to lead, guide or teach; to hold someone's hand and guide them through an illness. I was moved that this quintessential doctor should be the person who told me the quintessential meaning of his gift.

Hermes' staff, the caduceus, is the symbol of Western medicine, and the gifts of Hermes are related to medicine, including, as Zoë Playdon writes in *Medicine's Original Psychodrama*: 'the exercise of professional judgement, living with uncertainty, minute by minute, hour by hour, staying open to sudden changes, coping with twists and turns, and still finding the best route to health and wholeness for each individual patient. It is Hermes the compassionate Imagination who is the guide within the clinical encounter, drawing out the patient narratives and the doctor's responses.'

Manic depression is a tricky illness and people feel (and are) in a place of danger. My doctor gave me a sense of utter safety and protection, of being, in that tender phrase, 'under his care'. I had a kind of fantasy sometimes that he'd just wrap me up in a tartan blanket and put me in his pocket for a few months and then, in time, I'd be okay, with the osmosis of a kind, sane mind.

There was him, there was me, and there was a third place, the place between, where I could take my helplessly fluttering mind and huddle, safe, holding tight to the rope. He was 'there for me' in that simple phrase of pure gold. He made himself available, reachable. A couple of times, I felt I couldn't wait for an appointment and wrote scrawled messages for him which I left at reception. A couple of times I phoned. Each time, he responded, and fast. He didn't shunt me off to the circus of serial strangers which so many psychiatric patients experience, and I was grateful for that to the bottom of my heart. He was the NHS at its best.

'We ought to take pride in the fact that, despite our financial and economic anxieties, we are still able to do the most civilised thing in the world – put the welfare of the sick before every other consideration,' said Aneurin Bevan, father of the NHS. Meanwhile, during that awful year, when I saw my doctor for dozens of appointments, the Tory prime minister was suggesting that people should have just one free doctor's appointment per year. 'If the Tories get in again,' my doctor said with real feeling, 'there'll be no NHS.'

The mind, in manic-depressive breakdown, is precarious, fallible and mutable. It swoops, soars and slips. Flight collides with fall and the falls are brutal, breaking, bruising. But even the falls do not stay still. Cadences glitter in false certainty – 'all that is solid melts into air' – and the upswings run glissando arpeggios through you. Wherever I was, he positioned himself as a counterweight. When storm clouds overhead transformed to skylarks and I was flying, he gave me a sense of earthedness, holding a cautioning steadiness against mania. When firm ground turned to water under my feet and I was drowning, then he was buoyant and firm with gentle positivity. Both the drowning and the flying could reverse in minutes; flying fish and diving birds flickered from form to form, Escheresque, gold and blue, an amphibious either-air, an aether-ore.

Madness is frightening but, into the chasms of fear, he threw ropes of reassurance which I remember, even though I know I have forgotten much that happened in the first weeks. 'You *will* be okay,' was one of the few things I can remember my doctor saying in the early appointments. I felt as if I were hauling a memory of reason within me to try to hear this, because it took enormous discipline and willpower not to lose myself into the chaos unleashed in me. He repeated his reassurance hundreds of times over the numerous appointments I had with him, and he seemed to believe it so completely that I held to it like a lifeline. The confidence (or lack of) which a doctor feels about a patient's recovery can affect the outcome of their illness, probably never more so than when it is psychiatric in origin. 'You're going to be okay, you're going to be okay,' was unforgettable as a spell. It engendered belief in me and that belief went a long way to working its own cure.

In the week when Robin Williams, himself manic depressive, committed suicide, the media re-told the story of a young man, Jonny Benjamin, who was deeply depressed and about to jump from Waterloo Bridge. He was talked down by a passer-by. The point the passer-by made was simple and powerful: 'You will get through this.' No one, Jonny said later, had ever told him this before.

I held on to my doctor's confidence like a saint's relic and when I was alone I repeated to myself over and over his reassurance that I would get well. If he lost his confidence in himself or in the medication or in my recovery, he never let it show. I trusted him so I believed in his judgement; he said what he meant and meant what he said. I trusted him in another way, too: I confided in him, and felt that I could give him my hurt and secret things.

I had trusted him from the very first appointment I'd had with him, several years previously, not in a state of hypomania but of severe depression. During the three months prior to that very first meeting, I had spent weeks intolerably isolated, mainly sitting on the stairs, en route to the unreachable kitchen or the equally unreachable bed. I eventually made an appointment, walking into his office with some almost-but-not-quite-fictitious ailment, unable to say anything about depression. He dealt swiftly with this semi-fiction. Then he slowed right down, and I felt him searching my face. He asked what I did for a living.

– I'm a writer.

There was a pause.

– That must be very lonely.

Five words.

I wept and wept. The loneliness of my writing life, which fed the shrieking isolation I felt in depression, was named aloud. In five words, it was spelled and dispelled. Five words which began to link me back to the unlonely world. Five words which released me into being able to talk to a doctor about depression for the first time in my life, although I'd suffered from it since I was twelve.

In the intervening years, I'd seen him several times, and I felt he knew me in wellness as well as in illness. He had a yardstick to measure both the heights and depths of this current episode. Without that prior knowing, what does a patient face? What can a doctor do? A patient may need to explain who they've become, in depression, just when they are sinking to silence. They may want to portray who they truly are when they are well, just when that seems an unrecoverable state of grace. A doctor, meanwhile, attempting in ten minutes to diagnose someone they've never met, is working blindfold, sticking the tail on the donkey. Both of them often end up meeting in the no-man's-land of typical symptoms and the prescription *du jour*.

In the years between my very first meeting with my doctor and this Grand Madness, I had also used the placebo effect; if a person is ill, and they make a doctor's appointment, studies show they often begin to feel better simply because of having the appointment. So from time to time in those intervening years, if I was feeling shaky and low, I would make an appointment with him, and let the placebo effect work, and then cancel the appointment three days before.

John Berger wrote one of the most stunning books about the life of a GP, *A Fortunate Man: The Story of a Country Doctor.* 'Clearly the task of the doctor . . . is to recognize the man. If the man can begin to feel recognized . . . he may even have the chance of being happy.' In some cases, Berger writes of Dr Sassall, 'he faces forces which no previous explanation will exactly fit, because they depend upon the history of a patient's particular personality. He tries to keep that personality company in its loneliness.' This is a perfect rendition of the reason why my doctor was so curative for me. He kept me company in my loneliness. He *saw* me. He also saw where I was in this illness. There is a healing power in truth, sheer healing in honest appraisal, with nothing hidden, and he was candid. 'You're very fragile,' he said several times; other times he variously remarked: 'You've been very bad'; 'You've been in dangerous territory'; 'I've been very worried about you.' Those observations made me feel unalone. He was alongside me, and truly acknowledged where I was. In Berger's words, a good doctor does more than treat patients: he is 'the objective witness of their lives . . . the clerk of their records'. By witnessing and then naming aloud the situation I was in, my doctor made it at once real and recoverable.

I felt he was completely on my side and also wholly present; it felt as if he brought his whole self to the appointments, and this was equalizing. My mind had cracked open, been riven, wounded, horribly exposed. If I'd had to see a doctor who was masked, defended or guarded, who played a role or who wasn't truly present, it would have felt unfair, creating a power imbalance I would have hated. In madness, anything which increases one's sense of weakness and vulnerability is detrimental.

My doctor also openly acknowledged medicine's limits in dealing with the mind and yet made me feel he was not out of his depth. (Many of my friends were, and said so, and while I appreciated their honesty it left me feeling in greater danger. I was completely out of my own depth, after all.) I needed to feel I was in safe hands, and I was.

He could be funny and serious; he combined sensitivity with solidity. He was tact incarnate when he needed to be but could also apply blunt common sense. He also knew how to use the gears: when to move quickly and when to go very slowly. He simply *could* not have had the time he made for me: the hours, the late-running and over-flowing appointments. But he gave me – in his leisurely thoughtfulness, his unhurried manner – the impression that no time was unexpandable, no appointment unstretchable, that time and hurry and pressure and workload and speed were all a mild irrelevance which could be left in the waiting room with the forgotten umbrellas and the fluffy dinosaur. And yet the speed he used when he needed to was remarkable: first getting me on antipsychotics and later getting me to hospital when I could no longer see.

As the lead climber is just ahead of you on the mountain, so I felt he was just ahead of me in this crisis. When I was flailing around trying to force myself into recovery, impatient and angry with myself for all I could not do, he gave me wiser counsel, permission to be ill, repeatedly saying that, if I'd broken my leg, I'd have no problem accepting that I couldn't use it properly. A broken mind takes far longer to heal. Just as importantly, when the time was right, he gave me the encouragement and, more precisely, the expectation to be well.

At one point during this whole episode, I talked to one of my nephews about my doctor. My nephew usually has the sweetest temperament, but he became exasperated with me for the first time in his life.

'You're talking about him like he's a god or something. He's not a god. He's not a saviour. He's *just* a *man*. He's *just* a *man*. He's *just* a *man*.'

Three times. The vehemence of his tone drew me up short. We are very close and he understands me well. If he was upset, I knew there was matter in it. It was only later, when I read Darian Leader's *Strictly Bipolar*, that I could contextualize those feelings. Leader writes of manic-depressive patients idealizing their doctors: 'Pages of disappointment with mental health workers and medication will almost invariably be followed by a sentence such as: "Then I met the best doctor . . ." ' Leader surmises that 'it is not simply the doctor or the drug that has helped her but the actual function of idealization itself.'

Quite so, I thought, reading this. There you go. It's just a feature of being bipolar. I felt, as I did so often reading Leader's book, a sense of comfort in comprehension of the tricks and treats played on me by this condition, and there is, in my view, no other book which gives such a succinct and accurate portrait. And, at the same time, when I came to reconsider the question whether or not my doctor was a saviour, I have to say yes, he was: he saved my life. Was he an angel for me? Absolutely. I saw his wings.

I could 'see' the wings of people only very rarely, but every time was when I felt they had sent their minds in flights of under-standing to try to find mine. They could hear what I was saying and in turn, when they spoke, their words had the power to reach me. All of them could fluently speak a winged language, though accented according to their natures and the character of my rela-tionship with them.

All of them had minds which were fleet, kind, exact, close and precise. Like, I cannot help thinking, Wim Wenders's guardian angels in his film *Wings of Desire*, which describes a vision of a world in which we are surrounded by angels. Children see them. Angels recognize each other. Libraries are full of them.

I could see their wings when I had the strongest sense of an exchange, a commerce of comprehension which left me infinitely less lonely. When, in other words, they were being good messengers – and this is Mercury's doing: the winged messenger bringing images of wings. Part of the intensity of my gratitude is because they were willing to cross over into my sky – to risk the different temperatures and air pressures. They also gave my psyche strength, because it seemed to me that the touch of their wings in my mind suggested that perhaps I could even follow their flight down from the savage mountain into a meadowsweet valley – that perhaps I could trust their wings when my own were broken bits of sky made of stars as brilliant as stars are useless, scattered and disconnected across a cosmos of chaos and night.

Why wings? Because we fly, we humans, all of us, in thought, imagination and empathy. Not for nothing is Psyche winged, not for flight after death but for flight before death. Perhaps the human mind's age-old sense of angels arises from an insight of what is now called madness: the word 'angel' comes from the Greek *angelos*, meaning 'messenger', and in highly sensitive states the mind is quick to note the messages, hyper-alert to the transactions at the border between the outer universe of the world and the inner universe of the mind.

The idea of the angel seems the very force that drives poetry, the spirit of Orpheus, something which Charles Lamb understood, describing Coleridge as 'an Archangel a little damaged'. Angelism (as an idea within poetry), famous in Rilke's work, is a term said to have been coined by French philosopher Jacques Maritain, while the Portuguese scholar Eduardo Lourenço described poetic angelism as the practice of poetry where the angel stands as a metaphor for poetry itself, and for the driving force of *Logos*, the Word.

Wings, flight and feathers have a long association with the poet-seer tradition, so Hebrew shamans would chirrup like birds when they worked. Ireland's chief poets traditionally wore official robes made of bird feathers; court jesters wore a feather as part of their costume; and shamans around the world wear, or carry, feathers.

Angels and messengers like the Trickster can cross the border between inner and outer, between self and other; the messenger can transform, shapeshift, metamorphose, play the enigmatic role, occupy the quixotic space – genie, Ariel, bird or angel – and the moments when I saw people's wings were all when their psyches were inter-intelligent with my own, and I felt as lucky to have them around me as I would guardian angels.

'I WANT TO DIE,' I wrote in my notebook, in capitals of capital punishment.

It is a truth of mixed-state hypomania that you live at the poles: angels and demons, heaven and hell, levity and gravity dovetail with each other, while a sickening seesaw hurls you from one to the other. The major key becomes minor with just one chord-note altered. So it is that one moment I could be keeling over with laughter at something and then, in a delirium of pain, I could have happily driven off a cliff with a flick of the wrist, or jumped heedless as hopscotch under a fast train.

It was nearly midnight. In all senses.

It was 11 p.m. on December 21st, and I was in anguish. I wanted to read John Donne, who, incidentally, wrote the first defence of suicide to be published in English. As Donne wrote of this day, the shortest in the year, "'Tis the year's midnight, and it is the day's.' And it was mine. It was my midnight, mind benighted by itself. My life had set. To longest night.

I had had an appointment that day with my doctor but, with Christmas intervening, I wouldn't be able to see him for a week. The lifeline felt too insubstantial when it had to rope together days which were just too far apart. Its strength was whittled by time to a frayed thread. In that day's appointment, I despaired of my stupidity, because my doctor was saying the same thing – the same *right* thing, be it said: that I would get better and needed to take the medication. But this day I couldn't follow his leading. This day, despair flooded up in me. Suicidality engulfed me, and I began thinking seriously about doing a long-distance walk around the Welsh coast because in this flinty winter weather I could 'fall' off a cliff without much effort and with no explanation required. No *apologia pro vita mea*. This idea had been at the back of my mind for some weeks, but on this solstice night suicide tolled, hollow, low, now.

I didn't take the medication that day. Despair and alcohol got there first, and though a couple of friends were trying to persuade me, I refused. And there it was, suicide, no longer like a tormentor outside me but inside me, coiling around my heart, manipulating my mind. I did nothing other than a kind of silent keening for an hour. And then at midnight I picked up the telephone and phoned a friend. Asleep. Another. Same. A third, and I was praying: please pick up the phone. I have a friend who is an author and journalist, a man of great kindness but also, crucially, one of those people with a willingness and ability to take charge in difficult situations and an alertness to urgency and danger. Most of all, at this moment, his words had power for me, his voice a strong authority. He could outshout the suicidal callings – and he did.

Modernity can be obsessed with people expressing their feelings, spelling out their troubles and traumas, and conventional wisdom maintains that, when people are suicidal, they need to talk to some-one. But it seems to me that sometimes people who feel suicidal do not need to talk so much as to listen, because they need to hear a voice stronger than the siren voice of suicide. In the terrifying abyss of suicidality and severe depression, what a person may need is not a listening ear as much as a speaking voice, talking from a place of wellness, clarity, strength and confidence: life coming towards you. Someone whose voice can reach you when you are the pelican in the wilderness, ugly, inept, unwordable, silent except for those gut-croak cries for help.

– What about your nephews who you love so much? my friend asked. Your brothers? (One of my brothers, in America, who hadn't known about my suicidal feelings, rang me the following day and told me that on that same night he'd had his first ever suicide night-mare; something alien was ripping his guts out.)

– What about your friends who love you? You don't have the right to cause us such pain, he said.

More than anything, he appealed to my writing self.

– Your work needs you, he said.

I had been trying to explain to him that I didn't want to take medication because it would interfere with the glorious glimpses from the tops of the mountain, the sense that I could reach something of the mind's deeper insights if I only had the courage to stay in the mountain ranges.

– So you're doing this for your writing? he asked, double-checking.

– Um, yes, I said lamely.

— And how will you write if you're dead? I mean, forgive me for stating the obvious, but this is more than illogical.

It was, of course, mad.

He used a term I'd never heard him use before. Staying alive, he said, is a *sacred duty*. Then slowly, carefully, calmly and kindly, he simply told me what to do, utterly practical, in that voice stronger than the suicide voice. He told me to take the medication while he stayed on the phone. I did. He told me to find my cats and get them tucked up in bed with me. He told me to go to sleep and he'd call in the morning. He has my gratitude for life.

The figures for suicide in hypomanic mixed states are appalling. Twenty per cent. One in five. You feel low enough to want to and manic enough actually to have the energy. Being in a hypomanic mixed state carries the highest suicide risk of all mental illness.

People with manic depression are twenty times more likely to commit suicide than the rest of the population and, according to Andrew Solomon, author of *The Noonday Demon*, manic-depressive illness is the second-leading killer of young women. Kay Redfield Jamison notes that nearly half of those with bipolar disorder will try to kill themselves at least once and also writes that in manic depression 'any combination of symptoms is possible, but the one most virulent for suicide is the mix of depressed mood, morbid thinking, and a "wired", agitated level of energy.'

People with manic depression die sixteen to twenty-five years earlier than the average population. In mixed-state hypomania, a person can reel between suicide and the purest life force in minutes, as Mahler experienced, as he wrote to a friend when he was nineteen: 'The fires of a supreme zest for living and the most gnawing desire for death alternate in my heart, sometimes in the course of a single hour. I know only one thing: I cannot go on like this . . .'

'Shield your joyous ones,' says the Anglican prayer. 'It is a curious request to make of God,' notes Kay Redfield Jamison in her book on mania, *Exuberance: The Passion for Life*. Shield your joyous ones: for there is a terrible vulnerability in them, the high-risk skaters on thin ice.

In mountaineering, people talk of the 'death zone' (over 26,000 feet, or 8,000 metres; the peak of Everest is in the death zone, for example), where there is so little oxygen that the body cannot survive for long; climbers may reach into the zone for a short time but cannot spend too much time there. It was a perfect metaphor, for in this madness my mind was running out of the oxygen of sanity. In the death zone, my judgement was awry and I clung to the Voice of Reason, which spoke through my friends and through my doctor. The Voice of Reason was, I knew rationally, the one to heed. Sometimes I could see for myself that the world was just too beautiful to leave, but the howling pain drove me to de-say myself, seeking to be unspoken and unsaid, wanting obliteration, my voice annihilated. Suicide had a surly splendour to me then: sullen as depression, magnificent as mania. In moods of depression I was de-voiced, but in manic moods suicide seemed an expression of voice, a form of communication, an act of theatre, a swansong flung to Earth. Not a 'dead end' but an exaggerated performance, responding to life with a corresponding electricity: death. Suicide felt like a work of art, a flourishing, vital score, a blazon fanfare at the end of a symphony.

In depression, suicidality came to me with dulled despair, but in mania it came shining. It was oddly vital and extraordinarily appealing, as if my life could speak to Life only by *fucking* it, Eros–Thanatos in deadly embrace. As if, through suicide, I could have sex with the elemental life force, turn myself back to carbon again so the whole rolling life force could throw the dice for another turn.

Orgasm, of course, has been called *le petit mort*, the little death, as if sex contains a little seed of death. Likewise, in long cultural understanding, death contains a little seed of sex. I could be joined to Life by one stupendous death, an uproarious explosion, the eruption of a volatile volcano. Agony and ecstasy were on kissing terms; their lips hot, not to exit this individual life but to enter more deeply into Life itself, exorbitant and priceless. In manic mood, suicide seemed almost celebratory, an intoxicating temptation, an audacious, flagrant dare. It had primed me, flirted with me and thrown fizzing stars across my path. It had put the glitters on me.

In the extremis of this crisis, nothing could bear the weight of my emotions or withstand their temperature: as if fire had the weight of brute metal and my mind was a rolling ball of burning lead, and suicide was standing, like Hephaestus the blacksmith, working the boiling metal to the end-point of intensity.

Mixed-state hypomania is always on the move, it demands to go further, faster, higher, deeper; it has its eyes on the ultimate, the ultima Thule. Like fire, the more it burns, the more it will burn; it demands fuel and, if that is not freely given, the fire will grab what it wants, always onward, and in its heights as well as (more predictably) in its depths, it asks: Where to from here, except a blazing, euphoric pyre?

What surprises me most, looking back, is how mania caused a slippage in categorization. Suicide seemed as if it would be a momentary event without effect. It ceased to have import or corporeality; rather, it was a trivial, impetuous, reckless thing. *Reck*-less, it did not reckon; did not, and could not, count the costs. I wanted to feel disembodied, as if I could shuck off life and make my body a casualty of a casual tragedy. The casual way I thought about it frightens me now, but it was of a piece with mania's meanings. 'Casual' includes in its meanings both chance and accident: and we glimpse the signature of Mercury – in the realm of chance, we're in the territory of the Trickster.

I felt that life was something I could toss away like a spent cigarette. I could chuck it in the bin like an unwanted sandwich. Life or death seemed almost a question of housework: a bit of a sort-out. Keep it or throw it out? To be or not to be? Trash or treasure? It is the absolute opposite of Dignitas, that serious, real, considered, intelligent, planned, thoughtful dying.

After that first suicidal night, my friends seemed to link up, and made an unofficial rota so that I was never alone for long. I felt I was being parcelled around, from one house to another, or, if I was at home, there was a steady, regular pattern of phone calls. Even my friends who had never met got in touch with each other, swapped phone numbers, linked arms so I was in a silk net of care. It was sweet, touching and necessary. If I hadn't been so ill, I would have been embarrassed to be babysat like this. But I was, so I wasn't.

Christmas was hideous. I spent the day with friends and their kids and I was sky-high all morning. By lunchtime, I was in slippage. I adore children and I'm not normally irritable, but my nerves were shot to pieces and the children's noise and nonsense were making me want to shriek. The sound of Christmas champagne corks popping, normally one of my favourite sounds in the whole world, made me startle violently. Within half an hour I was lying in bed, my whole spirit aching, trying not to scream.

At my next doctor's appointment, I told him about the suicide night, but I needed to bring him something funny, too, so I told him about the time when Byron was seriously suicidal. 'I should, many

a good day, have blown my brains out,' he wrote, 'but for the recol-
lection that it would have given pleasure to my mother-in-law.'

Some of a doctor's work, my GP said, is to understand. Something physical – angina, for example – is easy. The psyche is harder
and takes a long time. We talked about suicide. Like my friend, my
doctor recalled me to my writing. Like my friend, he used the same
term: *duty.*

– What you have is a gift which is also a duty: a gift that demands
a heavy price.

My own mind had become unfamiliar territory. My brain, sleeping so lightly for so long, felt like a messenger in flight, travelling
light, carrying hand luggage only. I was a volatile insubstance.

Mania is like the high seas, calling the seafarer to set sail; it is an
enticing dare to the Odysseus within, who, hearing the siren call
and ignoring the whirlpools and rocks, embarks on epics. The siren
voices played me, swung me, seduced me; they wove harmonies of
beguiling danger, whispered me to whirlpools of suicidal spirals,
crafted their sway to lure me on to the rocks. Almost the last time
I drove, before I banned myself, I had ignored a T-junction sign and
driven recklessly right across the path of an oncoming car: it could
have been fatal.

I heard music differently, and it was as if I was not listening outwards towards the music but as if the music were already in me; it
was inside my psyche because its origin was in the universal human
mind. From there, it could be released by composers of genius, so a
song which had pre-existed in silence would be sung out loud for
the first time. For music transcribes mind. It is as if composers can
light a candle and step over an inner threshold and see by that
candlelight visible caves and cathedrals of the human psyche, and can
write the notes to describe it. I say visible, yet this is music and

therefore audible. But it felt to me as if music was in itself a profound synaesthesia (only connect); from its sound, music allows you to see. What chimes, rhymes and resonates (be it music, poetry or empathy) is curative; the mind is understood.

I wanted to breathe in the inspired air of Bach. Respiration as inspiration. What is to me the spire of song (Allegri's 'Miserere') is the irresistible aspiration within the psyche, for God or love or Orpheus.

Music, neutralizing the power of the siren song, is at the heart of the Orpheus myth. Orpheus sails with the Argonauts and, when they are in danger of being bewitched by the sirens' beautiful, fatal music, Orpheus draws out his lyre and plays music louder and love-lier than the siren song, and the ship sails safely on. It is as if Orpheus stands for the soul of music, and this story illustrates music's power over the psyche's self-destructions. If the siren voices of suicide seduced me, listening to music could sometimes swing me back round to safety.

It was a shock to hear music as I did at that point. Nothing could ever be quite as intimate as this when something from outside could steal gently into my psyche. The intensity of this intimacy is at one moment exquisite but might at a further pitch become unbear-able because it unveils part of the mind, usually curtained even to itself. It is utterly intimate, and yet music could hardly be more public; it happens, after all, in the fundamental commons of the air. Con-necting, linking the outer and the inner, it is part of the sense of connection which is key to mania. Hyper-connected, the manic mind is looking for rhyme and rhythm, sending out its lines into the world and responding in turn to the strings and cords and chords of strings. Unsurprisingly, composers, dwellers at that dangerous interconnect-ing border, suffer disproportionately from manic depression.

I did not just listen to classical music; Arcade Fire's flaming honky-tonk lit me sometimes, or Tom Waits would step into an evening with his raw, hurt hope, his self-bewildering, damaged brilliance, unfurling a gutterful of aces. But mainly I was tuned to classical. Sometimes I felt as if music painted the mind's sweetest serenity cerulean, sky blue and soaring, and I would feel like flying. *Tie me to the earth when the sky is so canted.* Tilted by its own incantatory song, world, stepping ever further inwards, becomes self. I was enchanted. Etymologically and actually. Bewitched by song – chant – which fascinated me and held me spell-bound, bound to listen, unfree to leave, surrendered to song.

Music created grandeur, the fullness of a composer's mind so august, so augmented, so matured, so autumned, that its golden chords swell to a ripeness so perfect there is no listening left for anything less, but then its gold gives, gives, gives into a sunset so blinding that in its grandeur, too, it becomes unbearable.

Sometimes I didn't dare listen to music, because I thought I would be lost; I'd never come back. Specifically, I thought if I really listened I'd never *eat* again; as if madness turned music to manna from heaven and if you've eaten the food of the gods you would never want mortal food again. Sometimes I would be frightened that music would mean a kind of dissolution, as if my words, my thoughts and my self-hood were made of sand and the inrush of liquid music would dissolve me entirely; no particularity would stand. All that would remain would be the rounded nubs of damp sand on a beach after the first wave has unspecified the sandcastle, and has departicularized the sharp, dry towers into soft, wet mounds. Then, lost to the tide and the tide's song, I would become music. What was 'I' would be gone.

The rest would be silence. Music wanted me, swamped me, took me and lost me, until, and finally, nothing more could be said. An ultimate creation of music is the quality of silence it inspires in the moment when it has ended – in Mahler's Ninth, for example – as the ultimate creation of a human life could be regarded as the quality of appreciation after its death. But the silence, perfected, exquisite, eloquent, is also unbearable because it silenced me. My words would die in the air, heaven too sweet for words or birdsong and therefore heaven unbearable for want of the imperfect, the twig that scratches, the awkward flit, the shadow that marks the afternoon, as if Earth is charged with the task of offering resistance to a perfect plainsong paradise.

When I found it hard to speak or, worse, hard to think, I played the piano. Sometimes I felt that it was descriptive playing – I played myself outwards, describing myself to the world, but this could go wild, as I played faster than my fingers could manage until, in the third movement of the 'Moonlight Sonata', the arpeggios ran to chaotic breakdown, a pile of notes spilling out of the keyboard's grip, falling scattered on the floor like a cascade of jackstraws, impossible to recollect. Sometimes I played like a kind of emotional blood-letting, to let out an excess of sadness or joy, to let it bleed out through the keys and into the absorbent air, until I played myself empty, but this tipped me into a barren loneliness, the self unecho-located in music.

There were moments when I played better than I ever have in my life, precisely because I could step over, into the music. The notes were in me like laughter before it is born into the world, like thought before it is formed in words; the melody was in my fingers already, only wanting a cue, a key signature, to begin.

The philosopher Susanne Langer in the 1950s suggested that music doesn't so much represent emotion as mimic it. If it mimics

84

emotion, it can surely also guide emotion, lead it, conduct it. The seventeenth-century musician Werckmeister theorized that well-crafted counterpoint was linked to the ordered progression of the planets, to the harmony of the spheres. At best, music harmonized me, it put the planets in order in my psyche, harmonized the hemispheres.

Most of the time, though, music-less, my brain felt like a jumble sale, stories unravelling like jumpers, torn quotes for 50p, a tatty memory, a broken joke, bits of thought, shreds of mashed paper, a malfunctioning processor, a tilted cabinet of shoddy files.

I blame Mercury. The rascal. In his footlooserie he was kicking up logic like leaves in the heels of his fast, feathered flight.

PART THREE:

THE TRICKSTER OF THE PSYCHE

All the old gods were aspects of mind, personifications of psychology, if you like, and Mercury is surely the god of manic depression. He has sneaked into language when we say someone is mercurial, the ancient Greeks and Romans intuiting something of the workings of the mind, for 'mercuriality' is the perfect word for the volatiles, those who fly too high and swoop too low, wings at their heels.

So Mercury flirted with me, intoxicated me and intrigued me. He seems to personify – with incredible precision – the features, character, experience and facets of manic depression. Mercury is known as one of the Trickster gods, and a huge number of cultures seem to acknowledge this very specific character. So widespread indeed is the Trickster figure that it leads me to suspect that it is in fact a code word for an aspect of the human psyche, recognized throughout history and across the world: and that aspect is tristimanic. That trickiest of conditions.

When you know what you're looking for, the sign of the Trickster is everywhere. He is there in fiction and in non-fiction, in the ancient texts and in sharply contemporary satires: he is there in Shakespeare, and in so many artists, writers and musicians.

But to Mercury, first. Even as a baby, Hermes 'has the look of a herald', we read in the *Homeric Hymn to Hermes*. Like a good messenger, he travels as well by night as by day; air or water or earth are equally his to cross. God of the Rizla packet used to catch a thought unawares or a scribbled phone number after a flirting night, Mercury carries crazy messages across the unhoused brain. For weeks of madness, Mercury had played my mind in the key of havoc; he won't come at my bidding but then arrives unannounced, the winged messenger, wings at his feet and his wrists, making mischief: a companion to no one except the falling, shooting stars.

Restless Mercury and reckless; even when the mind is all in order, he carries a high charge: he pours through you with the currents of Earth, he raises an electric storm in the brain. He galvanizes language, this god of metaphor and wit, yoking apart and splitting asides together. But when the mind is broken, Mercury grabs his chance, goes haywire, flicking the lights on and off, tripping all the switches. At the speed of light he makes connections between previously unconnected thought – he takes the corners too fast, jumps the gun, careless of what he drops.

This lean-to god stands on a slant, one foot uphill, cocky god, head on one side, tilted to the world. He travels light, he carries no weight and little power – he is the god who never asks you to kneel. Sometimes he is the god best honoured in the inattendance, glimpsed out of the corner of the eye; he is the last and least of the gods, after all, and he may reward you better in daydream than in watchful prose.

He is god of the crossroads, the roads between towns, god of benders, caravans and tents, god of tramps and trespass, border-crossing and waysides. But he is unpredictable, promising neither border control nor safe passage. Mercury as Trickster is the ruler of the in-between, the no-man's-land, the neither-nor. Way-farers pray to him and cairns are built for him, which is why his Greek counterpart is called Hermes, meaning 'he of the stone heap', described thus by Lewis Hyde in his fascinating book *Trickster Makes This World*: the cairn which is 'an altar to the forces that govern these places of heightened uncertainty and to the intelligence needed to negotiate them'. The cairn shows you your way, a guiding spirit to a path otherwise hidden, and sometimes Hermes-Mercury may be good to mountaineers and hillwalkers, to stop them being truly lost.

Mercury may offer cairns in the mind, too, when it has lost its bearings, or he may drive you madder, leading you astray with hallucinations of those spiral paths which I saw when I began to lose my mind, as if he were tempting me onwards towards a maze without a centre. When I was agitated beyond reason not to mislay scribbled messages to myself, Mercury teased me with lostness, for he is the god of the lost and found and hidden, god of lost minds and found friends, god of lost property, hidden beauty and found poetry, from the levity as 'snapper-up of unconsidered trifles' to the grave gravity of finding the soul in the underworld.

In terms of metallurgy, hidden gold is found by mercury, which adheres only to precious metals, so Mercury the god leads the way to the psyche's hidden gold. As guide of souls, Hermes fetches Persephone from the underworld, and the spirit of Hermes or Mercury travels between the ordinary daylight world and the deep subconscious of dream, instinct, metaphor and poetry, coming back with mind-gold as it comes back with mined gold.

Bringing Persephone back from Hades, Hermes hastens spring, and in a dark consonance of mind and season, it was the depth of winter when I was most ill, in what turned out to be the longest winter for fifty years. Spring will never come; Hermes has blithely forgotten.

Mercury-Hermes is the only shaman in the pantheon because he is able to go to the underworld and return: he moves between heaven and Earth, a knower of both the heights and the depths. He is at home in both eternity and time, life and death. In his rescue of Persephone, who was sentenced to live in Hades, one can read the narrative of manic depression as if mania, like Mercury the psycho-pomp, can conduct the psyche out of the hell of depression. Mercury has an element of anti-gravity, working against the grave of the underworld.

In fact, Mercury overturns gravity – he hurls you higher – Mercury, the only high-wire artist who doesn't care if he falls, because he can fly. He holds a candle for Icarus, careless of the wax-melt, because an ambition for wings is the signature of Mercury. In manic depression, if one cannot always walk, one can often fly. When it is hard to put on sensible shoes and walk through one's days in the ordinary working and waking world, yet one can fly in the unsensible fire flight. His feet as winged as his words, Mercury is agile, an escapee: 'ropes would not hold him . . . such was the will of Hermes,' we read in the *Homeric Hymn to Hermes*.

Of all the pantheon, he is the one whose energy quivers most fascinatingly: he is dynamic, quixotic, enigmatic. Fire is at the heart of him and Hermes is the inventor of fire, his character lit with magnetizing incandescence. 'Touched with Fire', that concisely perfect phrase of Christopher Isherwood's, was used by Jamison as the title of her outstanding work on manic depression and the artistic temperament. Both the Trickster Prometheus and Loki, the Northern European Trickster, steal fire. Manic depression, whose canting arms are fire and hurricanes, is often described in terms of flame;

flaring, sparking, lit, on fire. The Austrian composer Hugo Wolf remarked that in mania the blood becomes changed to 'streams of fire'. Mercury gives flame to the neurotransmitters so neurones can fire.

Hermes or Mercury (who tricks the more literal-minded Apollo) represents Imagination, as Zoë Playdon writes: imagination 'that not only sees newness everywhere, but brings it into being, demonstrated by his invention both of fire and of the lyre, both literal fire and the imaginative fire of creativity'.

Mercury jumps the gaps easily from unconscious to conscious, from night to day, because he is god of the gaps, the openings and rents. God of the intersections of roads, he is also god of the intersections of time. His hour is twilight, the no-man's-hour, as he is god of no-man's-land. Out walking at dusk, you search for the cairns as every day at twilight one looks for signs of significance – messages, news, stories – something feathered, fleet and lively; the ever-curious mind trying to see in the dark: what happens next? Mercury catches the hour of ambiguity and paradox, opaque and elliptical, and the deft mind, free of daylight jesses, is ownerless as an owl by night. The mind is its own twilight in its mercurial moments, every modality is twilit – it might be, could be, would be: the elastic hour stretched for its enigma and mystery. *Logos* sets its fixed ratios with the rational and setting sun. Mythos stirs and rises, cannier than we can ken at noon. Twilight reminds us every day that the psyche is a twice-dweller, fluent in languages intuited by night.

Hermes was 'born at dawn', and the Trickster is most active at the two joints of the days, dawn and dusk, when the light speaks twice; twilight is his time, he of the twins. Like the badger, he is twilight-striped, touched by two-light, day-streaked and night-stroked. At the last light and dawning dark, he stands silhouetted against the sky, a handful of light cupped in his west left hand. The Trickster relishes the twilight of the mind, the two-light of manic depression, the light-dark moments and, in the calling cadences of falling and soaring, the Trickster finds his flight.

Mercury is about when there is moonrise in the mind and the poet is listening, thinking the world by two-light, the actual and the metaphoric. There are no horizons to the mind, now, no limit to its insight. In the potent penumbra of twilight, human vision changes: our peripheral vision is actually better in twilight than in daylight, and this is both literally true and metaphorically true.

God of the periphery, god of the edges, Mercury is on the edge of the twelve Olympians, a margin-dweller in those margin hours of dawn and dusk. One hour in twelve is a twilight hour, the Trickster in the pack of hours, as Hermes or Mercury is Trickster to the pack of gods. The joker. A card sharp who plays his aces high but never plays by the rules. He is a double-dealer, a tricky one, and he can play nasty tricks on the manic-depressive mind, alluring you with a manic marsh-fire, wilfully leading you astray but dumping you stranded in a sump, the claggy mud of depression which he himself wouldn't touch with a bargepole.

Mercury has been called a generous thief – distracting me, he picked the pocket of my life, stealing a year. If he is a thief, though, he is a disarming one – an attractive one – and he gives as well as takes. Even when he is on the pilfer, he never takes everything; he will not steal all your savings, for he is the god of scavenged things, the overheard remark, the quixotic word; he knows himself to be the picker-up of priceless trifles. As he eavesdrops, he passes on what he hears, if he chooses: altering it if he feels like it, so you can never be quite sure.

Mercury, like all tricksters, is reliably unreliable. He plays Paganini to Saturn's Johann Sebastian: he plays a riff of extemporized brilliance in the cadenza then throws a wolf note to trip you up. He deals in luck, good or bad, but he never gives you your just desserts or pays his obligations. He is to be welcomed but never completely trusted: he knows where we hide our secrets and he'll spill them willy-nilly. Beware the quicksilver, for Mercury never minds his manners or his morals. He is a rogue, a rascal, an opportunist who fiddles the books, but he is not bad; he changes things for the better quite as often as he changes them for the worse. Integrity he has none: he is god of tegrity, how every thing touches another, and he leaves you touched by his visit; a little madder hatter with more mercury around the hat brim.

He is a messy lord of misrule and he plays a chaos croquet on a mole-heap lawn. He knows no duty of care but he will sometimes walk miles out of his way for you. A singular god of the unlinked, the surprising, solitary event, he is god of both serendipity and the non-sequitur –

The gap which lets a new conversation begin.

We say when a sudden silence descends on a party of people that an angel is passing over. People used to say that it was Mercury flying past. It is, in essence, the same thought, for Mercury is the messenger, which, as we've seen, is *angelos* in Greek.

The Trickster is Polytropos, turning many ways. Trickster is adept at transformation but also good at turning to new paths, he turns the page, writes the fresh chapter. Mercury, in alchemy, is a transforming agent by which base metals are transmuted, and Mercury is god of transformation, change and metamorphosis. It is the alchemy of art to translate, to spring the meaning from the trap of reality, in the quicksilver unlocking of poetry.

When the story is stuck, the Trickster moves it forward, jump-starting the conversation, oiling the wheels. But. He may equally just stop you in your tracks. He stopped me in mine when he tripped me up at Twyford Down. Mercury never sprains his ankle, his joints are winged where they articulate him. As messenger, he is 'articulate', and this word is connected to 'articulus', a joint in the body and a turning point in the year. And it was at the turn of the year that he tricked me badly: the winter solstice was the first of two nights when I became very suicidal, Mercury losing my reason on my behalf.

The Indo-European root behind the words 'articulate' and *articulus* is *ar*, which also gives us *arthron* (connection or joint). *Arthron*, meanwhile, was used by Aristotle to describe the connecting words of language, where meaning changes direction at a junction in a sentence, and the articulate Mercury is god of the intersections of thought. He is devious and deviating; his art is to connect and join, or to disconnect and disjoin. He is the hyphen in the sentence, connecting and holding apart. In the human body, he is god of the joints, and etymology is wise to this, showing us how the *ar-* root of Indo-European, which means 'to fit together or join', gives us the words for joints, *arthron* in Greek, *artus* in Latin; and, in English, a disease of joints, 'arthritis'. That *ar*-root also gives us the Latin word for art (*ars*) and English 'art' and 'articulate', the turning of thought into words. These words are cognate with *aša*, meaning 'truth' in Avestan (the language of Zoroastrian scripture). Keats would have been pleased.

Artists and writers are both blessed and cursed with Mercury's temperament, suffering disproportionately from mercuriality. He is a volatile substance, a fluent flame: a quickcyclist of moods. He doesn't like straight lines or concentric circles – he'll tickle the graph till the paper curls. But he raises merry hell as he does so, the old minds ruined, shafted by his sickness like Coleridge, or Byron taking the blame when it is Mercury who is mad, bad and dangerous to know.

He leaves his fingerprints everywhere on the pages of a life – he was reading under the bedclothes as a child, he demands that writers keep notebooks to catch an idea as it flies. Not for nothing is Mercury the god of writers and messengers. Shakespeare – as we'll see – has a very soft spot for him.

Mercury-Hermes and all tricksters have a special relationship with story, the writer's craft, names and their meanings, words and the roots of words, signs and the interpretation of signs. Hermes – god of signposts (always wise to notice, particularly at junctions) – was also god of speech, writing and interpretation, and he gives his name to hermeneutics, the art of interpretation. Part of the paradox of Hermes-Mercury is that his own signs are hard to read: he made himself shoes of branches – the branching thought, the dendritic connectivity of metaphor, is his domain – to hide his footsteps, as a poet may throw away the early notes, the steps by which a poem is made. So with Hermes-Mercury: his messages may be hidden but are treasured when found.

Hermes is a quintessential artist. He invented the lyre and 'lovely the voice that came from him' says the *Homeric Hymn to Hermes*. He sang of the gods and the Earth; he was the first poet. As Apollo listened, he was charmed and 'sweet longing seized his soul.' Apollo felt:

> *a deep and irresistible longing*
> *lay hold of his heart and he cried out,*
> *uttering winged words . . .*

. . . never before and by nothing else
has my heart been so moved.

A player in gift culture, Hermes is both gifted (talented) and gift-giving, making Apollo a gift of the lyre in exchange for glory. Apollo is intrigued by Hermes' giftedness – did it come from humans or from gods?

What art is this, what muse
for inconsolable sorrows,
what skill?

Mercury tricks and is tricked, he treats and is treated, as manic depression does. He is volatile, subversive, unruly and liminal; his thoughts fly, he gets high as a kite. This messenger-god danced a fandango with my brain's chemical messengers till Psyche tried to plead with him on my behalf to calm down a bit. But he was off, playing my mind, stealing the sleep of reason – in hypomania it is hard to sleep – and firing nightmares, waking me with brain fever.

Darian Leader includes among the key motifs of manic depression a 'large appetite, be it for food, sex or words'. Mercury, like all tricksters, is as libidinous as disinhibited mania; he is appetitive and hungry for meat and sex.

He disrupts the ordinary, sometimes positively, and sometimes negatively, for he is neither moral nor immoral but amoral. The Trickster Puck would 'mislead night-wanderers', and the words of the *Homeric Hymn* apply to Puck as much as to Hermes:

A few he helps, but he endlessly beguiles
the race of human beings in the darkness of the night.

98

He is there in the rolling drollery of Coyote, Native American Trickster. He throws the curve-ball and struts in the comic bouleversement of the clown; he is at the heart of flux, shift and swerve. He is the spin in the serve. The spice in the stew. The sudden skid. He is associated with traps, both releasing things which are trapped and setting traps and snares: often, though, he is himself caught in his own trap.

You probably know him in some of his guises: he is there in Malcolm Tucker, the spin doctor in the series *The Thick of It*. Wily and amoral, he is a tricky character who drives the action; articulate, funny, trapping people but ultimately caught in his snare: captivating and taken captive both. Douglas Fairbanks plays the Trickster in the silent movie *The Thief of Bagdad*, as the lascivious, attractive, slippery, mocking pickpocket. Trickster is there in McMurphy (Jack Nicholson) in *One Flew over the Cuckoo's Nest*, temperamental, mentally agile, clever, observant and funny. Like the classic Trickster of tales, McMurphy makes things happen; he unsticks the story, springs the trap, liberates others even though he is caught for ever in the trap himself.

Zorba the Greek, the exorbitant Zorba with his appetite for food and sex, his mischief and guile, is a perfect portrait of Hermes. 'His imagination laid traps for him and he fell right into them.' Amoral to the core, Zorba says, 'God and the devil are one and the same.' Zorba lies and cheats and charms: he is magnificently physical, with unbounded energy, and when he danced 'his feet and arms seemed to sprout wings.' Zorba is counterpointed by the Apollonian authorial voice, and they have a brotherly relationship. Like Hermes, Zorba plays music of such exquisite entreaty that the narrator-Apollo is moved, and in the very last sentence of the novel we learn that Zorba gives the narrator the gift of the santuri, as Hermes gave the lyre to Apollo.

In real life, the Trickster can be found among cartoonists and comedians, often divisive, communicative and brilliant, and indeed a force that forces a dialogue forward. He is there in the best kind of journalism: mischievous, deft, devilishly good at unpicking a locked politician. But the most significant Trickster of our age is Julian Assange. His first *nom de guerre* was Splendide Mendax, a name taken from Horace, meaning 'nobly untruthful', which precisely suggests the tricksy, unreliable, amoral character of a Trickster. Hacking is our generation's version of the lock-picking, trap-springing activity of the typical Trickster. Assange works on the borderlines of morality, ethics and politics, driven by an appetite which seems both egocentric and public spirited; he is famously unreliable, but it is impossible to gainsay his influence in the realms of communication and publication. He is the quintessential messenger, passing on millions upon millions of messages. He has often been in flight, literally and in terms of law: like the typical Trickster, it is an appetite for sex which seems to have led him into trouble. His action drove a million plot lines, forced forward a world-narrative of momentous significance. The fact that he utterly divides opinion between those who think he is a hero and those who think he is a nasty little narcissist is exactly the kind of split reaction the Trickster evokes.

You may have picked up a scent of the Trickster in the mad March hare, far from stupid but often unwise; wild, impetuous and hare-brained. Like Trickster, the hare is a changeful creature, moon-struck and associated with lunatic cycles. The hare is associated with fire and flight, with inventiveness and with artistic creation: a shapeshifting creature of lightness over weight (the levity of the leveret). It seems only too appropriate that the manic-depressive poet William Cowper kept tame hares. He described their different characters, but one of them in particular was exceptionally close to him and would let him pet it and carry it in his arms. It would fall asleep on his lap and, waking, would get him to take it into the garden by drumming on his knee or pulling on his coat.

Trickster is everywhere. In ancient Egypt, Thoth was a Trickster god, associated with the moon, wisdom and magic, and was the inventor of language and scribe of the gods: again the Trickster is associated with writing. The Trickster has something of the djinn about him; unstable, mutable, flowing as an arabesque. Shakespeare's Ariel, djinn-like himself, is a Trickster, both tricker and treater, neither mortal nor divine, creature of air and fire, charged with message.

Raven is a famous North Pacific Trickster figure; a glutton and a lech, he is nevertheless the dynamic principle of life, and in Haida creation myth he steals water and daylight. Raven teaches the first men some clever tricks, and they are adept learners, suggesting that humans may be the tricky addition to nature, the articulation of the world and its art; the trap-setters and the manipulators of nature, making hell and heaven both. Indeed, humans are the motive force which moves the story on, for better or for worse. Appetitive, clever and wily, mankind may, like the Trickster, set a snare but end up being the one caught in it. (The best example of this is, surely, climate change, where humanity, in a form of collective greed, is caught in its own trap and set to suffer its consequences, the monkey with its paw stuck in a jar grasping a nut, so greedy for the nut that it cannot drop the nut and release itself.)

If humans were seen as a trick played on nature, it seems to me that manic depression is a trick played on human nature: that amoral treat-trick hurling you heaven and hell, depression is a terrible trap, which snares you; mania may liberate you, but, in its disinhibition, it sets afresh a new trap to fall into. Mania fizzes around the mind, hyper-connecting at all the joints of art and articulacy, mouth open, words streaming out, while depression under-connects and snaps the trap shut. Author Michael Greenberg, writing of his daughter's mania, seems to reach unconsciously to Trickster imagery: mania seemed 'wily and insistent. It speaks to her in a whisper, promising riches, deviously finding a way to escalate and live on.'

Trickster is speedy, as one is speedy in mania, driving too fast and talking too fast: Hermes 'leapt out' of his mother's womb, and 'did not lie still for long'. Trickster is strongly associated with luck, both good and bad. Gambling in all senses, he is a dicey, opportunistic character. He is 'genius of the gods and bringer of luck', says the *Homeric Hymn*.

The manic-depressive mind recognizes itself in other minds, in certain lines of poetry, in certain memoirs and descriptions. The drum, the glint, the grin, the brain in burlesque visited by a motley fool, emotions somersaulting in an acrobatics of merry-melancholy. This can be glimpsed out of the corner of the eye, in the zany, the joker, the harlequin, so often depicted in feathers and striped clothing: their variegated moods perfectly expressed in the strong contrasts of light and dark, the bipolar kit, half and half.

Meanwhile, if you half shut your eyes, you see that the sad clowns of our age are dressed in the same feathers (Mercury's heel feathers) for the flight of speech and mind. Robin Williams. Stephen Fry. Ruby Wax. Each stands alone. They are not herd animals of their craft but a Guild of Singulars, and yet comedians with manic depression come from an ancient and exquisite lineage: the inspired jester, announcing themselves with bells, not attention-seeking but certainly audience-seeking, giving it their all, in the munificent generosity of mania.

The figure of the jester is not the same as the poet, but they overlap in the wise fool, telling the deepest truths, willing to curse and to pray. The ancient figure of the cursing-poet, incidentally, seems to have an uncannily similar posture whether it is the Irish *glam dichenn* or the Arabic *hija*, according to literary scholar Enid Welsford, standing to utter curses 'on one foot, one hand, one eye'. One in each world. One foot, hand and eye in the real world, the other in the spirit world. And that is how many poets live: half in the real world, half in the world of metaphor, imagination and the old glamour of faerie.

The nineteenth-century scholar Paul Lacroix visited Versailles and found an 'old man living there, with white hair, surrounded by old furniture, old pictures, old knick-knacks and a multitude of relics in the fashion of Louis XVI . . . it was Marie-Antoinette's fool.' As Enid Welsford writes: 'Versailles, empty of its kings, had retained a court jester as a living ruin.'

And in our age, which has emptied itself of so much colour, has robbed the human spirit and left little but relics of a psychic splendour, it seems to me that we, the bipolar-mad of today, take the role of the unemployed court jester, crying for our demeaned status as living ruins when, in the remains of magic, mystery and majesty, we are reduced to pathology. If we do not have a role worthy of our *wōdness*, then we *will* be ill, for illness is the only category which our culture allows us in this age of literalism, of numbering and of unwonder which, in mass media above all, would destroy the human mind's Versailles and replace it with the architecture of brutalism.

How to parse the Trickster in the grammar of society? Ask Shakespeare. The captivating Mercutio in *Romeo and Juliet* was a man 'possessing all the elements of a Poet: high fancy; rapid thoughts; the whole world was as it were subject to his law of association,' wrote Coleridge. The very name Mercutio means 'related to Mercury', and what Coleridge saw in Mercutio was a mirror for Mercury and, indeed, a mirror for his own psyche. The speed, frenzy, punningness, prolixity and associativeness of Mercutio's character are mercurial and manic-depressive qualities. His dynamic physical energy dances and soars, it seeks exercise and sex; he is as rude, carnal and appetitive as any Trickster. His mind is in flight with the imagery of wings, in his jesting, leaping, free-associating thinking, connecting anything with everything. Though he is moody and irritable, yet his exuberance is infectious, for he is pure cadenza; the rising falls of mania course through him in air and fire. Mercutio is, like all Tricksters, a neither-nor character: being neither a Capulet nor a Montague, he can cross over between their two worlds. The Nurse calls Mercutio a 'saucy merchant', not a gentleman, and Mercury is god of merchants, commerce and transactions. Trans-actor himself, he is alive to border-states in all directions.

The Trickster is deftly portrayed in Shakespeare's Autolycus in *The Winter's Tale*. He is 'littered under Mercury', we are told: born in Gemini, twins of this bipolar twinning state. (The staff of Hermes, the caduceus, has two twinned snakes.) He is called 'a wily fellow' in Robert Greene, Shakespeare's source, like the cartoon Trickster Wile E. Coyote. The *Homeric Hymn* relates how even as a child Hermes was 'wrapped up in crafty wiles'; and Apollo calls him a rogue, Trickster and crafty-minded cheat.

This is him! I gasped when I thought about Autolycus. This is *Mercury*.

– Meet me at the crossroads, Mercury had said to me, and so I'd waited there, not knowing what would happen. Shakespeare happened.

At the crossroads of the mind. At the junction of writer to reader. At the intersection of time, which is the eternal present moment when Shakespeare speaks – always at the heart of now. For Mercury has dazzled many a mind before ours and the Trickster has tricked many a shepherd.

Autolycus is a hedge musician, a balladeer on the byways, following in the footsteps of the musical Mercury. Autolycus lives in his own world and within his own moral code. He needs society yet he operates as a sole trader, a soloist to the core, always on the edge, at the boundaries, and on the road, in the no-man's-land: liminal as any Trickster. Hermes is lord of the land of sheep and a cattle-rustler, while the name Auto-lycus means 'the wolf himself', preying on the sheep-people who surround him as he filches from them at the sheep-shearing. ('Sheep-shearing' was a term for conning people, as 'fleecing' still is.)

There is a word in French practically invented for Autolycus or, more widely, the Trickster: *voler*. It means to fly, to steal, to wing, to pick, to rip off, to filch, to fleece, to hook, to crook and to convey a message. Autolycus exemplifies these: fleet of foot, stealing, winging it when he needs, picking up the unconsidered trifles, ripping off the clown, filching purses, fleecing the rustics by hook and by crook and, above all, conveying messages. Volatility permeates his role and his nature.

Autolycus is a portrait of the artist as Trickster, albeit in a comically disparaging portrayal. 'My traffic is sheets,' he says, punning on the 'sheets' which he steals from washing lines and re-sells as ribbons, and the sheets of writing paper, which were expensive and precious. (It's quite possible that writers would steal them in hard winters to write their tales.) Another interpretation combines the two: Shakespeare famously nicked the 'sheets' of other writers, stealing the broad outline of their stories, cutting them to ribbons, making something far more precious and re-selling them. This is how Autolycus sells his ballads, as ribbons ripped off from larger sheets of plays, making him, quite literally, a rip-off merchant.

Autolycus is a past master of his art: 'I understand the business, I hear it: to have an open ear, a quick eye, and a nimble hand, is necessary for a cut-purse,' he says, and it is as true for writers in show business as it is for pedlars: it is Shakespeare who also needs an open ear, a quick eye and a nimble hand. Historically, the two professions were linked in another way: the Vagrancy Act of 1604 decreed that those who had no land, no master and no legitimate trade could be branded 'R' for Rogue. But, intriguingly, the act exempted pedlars and also liveried players, so while most people were subject to laws forbidding vagrancy, both a Shakespeare and an Autolycus were part of a fraternity of vagabonds allowed out on the byways, the roaming roads between towns, the Trickster places, as Autolycus sings: 'Jog on, jog on, the foot-path way.'

Autolycus is a petty thief and conman: someone who, in Elizabethan England, used wit and snares rather than brute force in his borderline criminality. In the gleeful amorality of a Trickster, he remarks: 'Though I am not naturally honest, I am so sometimes by chance,' and he is grandiose about any divine judgement: 'for the life to come, I sleep out the thought of it.' Like the Trickster he is associated with traps and we hear him whisper of the Clown: 'If the springe hold, the cock's mine.'

He is a rogue, yes, but not a heavyweight criminal. He steals the Clown's 'spice' money but not his entire livelihood. He nicks the cash for the bawdy spice-of-life stuff but, generous thief as all Tricksters are, he gives back far more than he takes and does so in the form of the art he brings, with songs and stories. Autolycus is the link (the joint, the connecting point) between worlds, between the court world and the country world, as Shakespeare himself was; a translator who could bring the country to the court. He offers himself as 'advocate', or messenger, for the shepherd in the traditional go-between role of Mercury-Hermes. He makes trans-actions, movements across borders, both in the petty ways and in the greatest: as a pedlar, making iffy financial transactions, Autolycus honours Mercury as god of merchants looking after commerce of all kinds; but Autolycus also effects the grandest transactions, dealing between the worlds of the living and the dead, between the first half of the play, with the 'dead' Hermione and Perdita left for dead, and the second half, where life springs back, the trap released. In the role of Trickster, Autolycus sets the action going when things are stuck, he moves the plot forward. (The same role which Shakespeare, as every author, must always play.) In this wintry story, iced and stuck fast, Autolycus enters, singing of spring, changing the temperature and altering the tone.

Like the typical Trickster, Autolycus is appetitive and greedy, vital, vivid, attractive and speedy. As befits a Trickster tale, messages and the speed of messengers are all-important. The Trickster can be a personification of chance, and when Perdita is abandoned she is thrown into the realm of chance, the lap of the Trickster, as Paulina speaks of 'the casting forth to crows thy baby-daughter': crows are the birds of Mercury.

In the first part of the play, Antigonus obeys the orders of the jealous king and abandons the baby Perdita on the coast of Bohemia. It is thought that the same actor who played Autolycus would also have played Antigonus, embodying the Trickster's two-in-one trick-and-treating nature. Antigonus loses Perdita, and Autolycus finds her: both finding and losing are under the auspices of Mercury. But there is more: Hermione's name is related to 'Hermes' and is said to mean 'a lucky find', and it is also interesting that as Hermes means 'he of the stone heap', it is to stone that Hermione is turned until the finding of her daughter turns the play back towards life, as the turning world rolls winter into spring.

Sometimes what is most important is to ask the right question.

In the legend of the Fisher King, the knight Percival has a chance of curing the sick king if he asks the one curative question: Whom does the Grail serve? In manic depression, the difficult question, but also possibly the curative one, is this: What does it *want*, this madness?

Language.

In my case, specifically, poems. But it wants language in all its forms, the language of words and the tongue, the language of the body and sex, the language of music, of gifts. I know when I'm getting dangerously high: it's when my dearest desire is to 'learn' Indo-European not as a source of ultimate etymological roots but almost as a language. (Flight of ideas? Grandiose plans, anyone?) I'm looking for both the *arkhe* and the *echt* of language, the primal, the basis, the arch-language and also the most specific, the most sharply delineated and defined. The language which connects the present with the past, the language which connects so many different languages to each other, the language which gives a depth of meaning to each word it remembers.

Language is a key feature of manic depression. Darian Leader notes: the 'verbal dexterity and sudden penchant for wit and punning', and he identifies, in all its simplicity, the medium of connectivity in the human world: 'it is language.' Depression, by contrast, is a kind of denotative language. It sees words flat, each word lonely, stubbornly unconnected, holding only one meaning. Puritan language. Black and white. No frills. But mania, delightfully, is a connotative language. It makes associations and friendships. It cannot walk alone but links itself lovely to others. It is playful language, seeking thrills, punning and suggestive; it loves a good *double entendre* as much as the next man.

Only connote, only connote . . .

Mania can connect everything with everything, because it is inquisitive to life and its senses are connected to the world. In manic mood, I felt connected to language, people, animals – even objects. Things came alive in my hands, so my notebook had a pitiful, mewing losability until I wanted to say to it: *Hold my hand when we're crossing a road.* My woodstove grinned, its shoulders heaving like a drunken old man trying not to laugh. My piano stretched itself like a luxuriously naked body, asking my fingers to play it into ecstasy. My favourite candlestick, a Wee Willie Winkie brass one, saw out the nights like a vigilant nightwatchman. It was as if the brass itself could become rubber, pliable and transformative; as if a piano could be made of elastic and stretch to my touch, the keys nibbling my fingers; and the whole world torrential with animation.

The brain connects and communicates with itself as neurones (brain cells) 'speak' to each other through neurotransmitters, or nerve messengers. Like a million million Mercuries in the brain, neurotransmitters are located at the junctions (like Mercury at the crossroads) where one neurone meets another. These junctions are called synapses, from *syn* (together) and *haptein* (to fasten, join, connect). God of the joints, mischievous connecter. 'Connect' is, effectively, the same word but in Latin rather than Greek: *con* (together) and *nectere* (to bind or tie). While mania is an over-connected electric charge, in depression the switch is flipped and the supply is disconnected. Nothing comes of nothing, nothing goes to nothing, nothing speaks to nothing.

If normal thought includes following a line of thinking as the feet walk an iambic pentameter along a drovers' way, in madness everything changes. Your mind has as many feet as there are infinitely discriminable points on a compass-rose. The psyche is centrifugal, not linear, and it blooms like the seed head of a dandelion. I felt I could think for miles in all directions at once.

Connections come in many forms, and social connections are created (or strengthened) in the language of gift, which, as Lewis Hyde so brilliantly describes in *The Gift*, are life-ful only if there is a sense of motion, so everyone must keep the cycle of gift-giving going round. But in mania, gift (and, indeed, giftedness) can be problematic, if touching. One person I know of with manic depression kicks off an episode by buying rounds of drinks, giving and giving until he is broke. A Timon of our times, he cannot afford it, but the Trickster has a hold of him, generous to others, though thieving from himself.

Seeking connection with others, many people with bipolar read the memoirs of fellow manic depressives to find companionship across the world and, indeed, across centuries. William Cowper wrote in *The Castaway*:

> But misery still delights to trace
> Its semblance in another's case.

For me, it is in Shakespeare that I most keenly seek to trace the resemblances of this condition because he understood manic depression and caught its exact signature over and over again. He littered his plays with little clues, so those who came after him, mad and manic and keening to be understood, desperate to find and be found, could gather up the clues like little pebbles in a fairy tale and find their way through the forests of the mind. In Shakespeare we can see our understander: in his work we can know that we are known. Why does Shakespeare matter so much to me? Because, in his presence, I can breathe in fully. The air which animates me, he anticipated. The words by which I live, he coaxed from language.

Mania, depression, or both, affect a large number of Shakespeare's significant characters: Mercutio, Antonio in *The Merchant of Venice*, Jaques in *As You Like It*, Hamlet, Lear, Timon and Cleopatra. The subject of moods and manias permeates specific plays, including *A Midsummer Night's Dream* and *As You Like It*. Shakespeare's love for puns and his genius for word creation, his sense of empathy and connection, his feeling for connotation and word association, his ability to say so much in so few words, all suggest that Shakespeare either experienced manic depression or understood it intimately in another. In his use of soliloquies, too, he shows the theatre of the mind (that most profound play within a play), particularly when that mind is disjoined from normal social interaction and dialogue.

We know it is common for writers to have manic depression: we also know it is an illness that asks for audience, a state of mind which is in itself a theatre; it is a communicating, messenger-driven state of mind.

Charles Lamb wrote: 'It is impossible for the mind to conceive of a mad Shakespeare,' but I would say that, while it is hard to think of Shakespeare writing while experiencing madness, it seems only too possible to conceive him writing after – or between – episodes. Shakespeare, in Sonnet 147, describes a feverish, dangerous lovesickness as an illness akin to what we'd now call manic depression.

The sonnet's protagonist loses his reason, seeing his thoughts and words 'as madmen's are', and interprets his beloved in acute polarity, angelizing and demonizing her; he is death-obsessed and sleep-deprived with reckless energy; of this Shakespeare writes five words which stand as a deft description of mania: 'frantic-mad with ever-more unrest'.

The word 'frantic' meant 'insane' from the mid-fourteenth century. From the late fifteenth century, it picked up a more specifically manic definition: 'affected by wild excitement'. It carries meanings of frenetic, frenzied, disjointed or chaotic, and was used later by William Cobbett, describing 'a man of violent and frantic disposition'.

In *Romeo and Juliet* Mercutio plays a burlesque spirit-messenger as he cries, staccato:

> *Nay, I'll conjure too:*
> *Romeo! humours! madman! passion! lover!*

In *A Midsummer Night's Dream* those terms have modulated from 'madman', 'passion' and 'lover' to 'lunatic', 'lover' and 'poet' – a threesome familiar to manic depression – as Shakespeare seems to find the common denominator of all three in the frantic frenzy of polarizing moods.

> *The lunatic, the lover, and the poet*
> *Are of imagination all compact:*
> *One sees more devils than vast hell can hold,*
> *That is, the madman: the lover, all as frantic,*
> *Sees Helen's beauty in a brow of Egypt:*
> *The poet's eye, in a fine frenzy rolling,*
> *Doth glance from heaven to earth, from earth to heaven.*

In part, this follows the Renaissance honouring of *furor poeticus* as Plato and Aristotle understood it: the madness of the poet, the mark of divine inspiration, the 'fine madness' 'which rightly should possess a poet's brain', in the words of Elizabethan poet Michael Drayton.

A Midsummer Night's Dream opens with a portrayal of the rational mind firmly in the world of flat fiat, predetermined lives and predictable laws, the Court of Athens, mean-lipped with its doling-bells, the world of judgement and the awful demand to be only part of yourself.

But it swiftly moves to show the mind's states where dream, imagination, passion, poetry and madness rule, and mania has its day: 'A calendar, a calendar! Look in the almanac; find out moonshine, find out moonshine!' We are in the world of Puck the Trickster, the 'mad spirit', wings at his heels, putting a girdle about the Earth in forty minutes, as fast as mania can trippily switch to depression. He guides and misguides, misleads people in his realm: 'I am that merry wanderer of the night.' When Shakespeare decided to give his lead female character the name Hermia, he was giving us the clue that we are in Hermes' Trickster territory, and the punning language is a constant reminder of the swirlingly irrational psyche, as when, for example, Demetrius describes himself as 'wood within this wood', where the first 'wood' means *wōd*, mad or frantic.

Looking, finding and seeing are themes of the Dream; eyes are crucial. The play conjures a way of seeing which is like the dizzyingly volatile world of mania. Everything is mutable. Puck is a shapeshifter; Titania has a changeling child; lovers alter their loves under an inconstant moon. Everything at every moment is springing, curling, unfurling, grimacing, gurning, clowning. Yet, like the faerie sleight of sight, you can't quite catch anything in the moment of its transformation, but rather you are aware, from the corner of your eye, that something shimmers and glistens, the play of light on water, a scent-shadow of bluebells at dusk, the essence of *escence*, as it were: something within the very process of its being: iridescence, effervescence, oscillescence, the beauty of instability. But then, imagination, having run riot and created havoc ('now are frolic'), makes its peace with reason at the end. Returning to one's normal self is like reawakening into the ordinary and looking back on an episode of madness: one sees it 'But as the fierce vexation of a dream'.

Many people who have known mania and hypomania have a longing for it; it has seduced them, and they miss it when it is gone. The Dream conjures precisely that sense of nostalgia for the mind in its less ordinary states; it reminds me specifically of the nostalgia for mania when an episode is over. Once one has been possessed, temporarily beguiled and bewitched, one may well want to return to the *wōd* woods but must re-enter the sensible Court of Athens, though always taking a peek back over one's shoulder to see if that naughty Puck is still playing a trick or three.

Antonio in *The Merchant of Venice* is a famous example of causeless depression arising of itself, but Solanio introduces the idea of bipolarity, swearing 'by two-headed Janus' and remarking the extremes of human nature, from the manic characters who would 'laugh like parrots at a bagpiper' to those who will not, cannot, smile.

Janus, the bi-psyche god, had one face which smiled and one which frowned, as if bipolar were etched in his image. (The jester's marotte, the head on the stick, would often be carved with the two faces of Janus.)

As You Like It locates polarities of temperament in the two people in fool position: Touchstone and Jaques. The name Touchstone is interesting: something which tests the true nature of metals and, equally, tests the true mettle of human nature, as manic depression seems to sound out and detest what is fake, untrue or inauthentic. The role of the jester, of course, is similar: a tester of the fake and a touchstone who has the privilege – and capacity – to speak home truths. Touchstone – merry, mad and wearing motley – represents mania. Jaques – melancholy, philosophizing and dressed in black – stands for depression, as the play notes:

> *Rosalind*: They say you are a melancholy fellow.
> *Jaques*: I am so; I do love it better than laughing.
> *Rosalind*: Those that are in extremity of either are abominable
>   fellows.

To my ear, these lines have the tone of an in-joke, suggesting accustomed exasperation on the part of Shakespeare or perhaps one of his players, knowing manic depression like a visitor: both familiar and (sometimes) unwelcome.

Of course, Shakespeare may have been abstractly curious about melancholy, known as 'the Elizabethan malady', and, of course, too, it may be the case that Shakespeare did not experience manic depression himself but, rather, closely observed others who did, perhaps including Robert Armin, his clever clown, who is thought to have joined Shakespeare's players in 1599 and given new depth to Shakespeare's fools.

'If any player breathed who could explore with Shakespeare the shadows and fitful flashes of the borderland of insanity, that player was Armin,' wrote John Leslie Hotson in *Shakespeare's Motley* in 1952. Add to that the fact that he was a solo comedian and a writer, thought to be the author of a pamphlet called 'A Pil to Purge

Melancholie', published in 1599, and it looks like Armin is seriously lining up the black, in terms of manic depression. Armin was by trade a goldsmith, giving resonance to his playing (and probably co-creating) the character of Touchstone, that tool of the goldsmith's trade. He also played Feste, Lear's Fool, the Porter in *Macbeth*, the Fool in *Timon of Athens* and Autolycus. Armin was fool-fascinated, exploring all aspects of clowning, interested in the 'philosopher-fool', the jester and the zany. He wrote about the distinction between a fool artificial and a fool natural, which delighted Ken Kesey (himself the creator of that fool natural McMurphy). A true fool natural, says Kesey, 'never stops being a fool to save himself; he never tries to do anything but anger his master, Sir William. A fool artificial is always trying to please; he's a lackey. Ronald McDonald is a fool artificial. Hunter Thompson is a fool natural.'

Hamlet is a portrait of the psyche at stress. Famously, Hamlet suffers nightmares, hallucinations, volatility, aggression and grandiosity, coupled with bleak misery as he thinks of suicide. These combined characteristics are an acute rendition of manic depression, though of course it is a moot point whether Hamlet is truly suffering madness or making a pretence of it. Shakespeare doffs his cap to Timothy Bright's *Treatise of Melancholy* (1586) as Bright writes that 'the air meet for melancholic folk ought to be . . . open and patent to all winds . . . especially to the South, and South-east,' while Hamlet says, 'I am but mad north-north-west. When the wind is southerly, I know a hawk from a handsaw.'

King Lear can be read as a portrait of manic depression. Lear is impetuous, speedy, agitated, excessive in generosity, poor in judgement, irritable, grandiose, and suffers hallucinations. Shakespeare, in setting part of the play in a storm, makes real a frequent metaphor of the manic psyche, that the onset of madness is like a storm and that the mind's metaphoric world surpasses the actual world in intensity and significance:

> *The tempest in my mind*
> *Doth from my senses take all feeling else*
> *Save what beats there.*

In lines which are heartbreakingly apt for anyone who has known what it is like to cross the threshold of sanity while retaining insight sufficient to fear it, Lear cries out:

> *O, let me not be mad, not mad, sweet heaven;*
> *Keep me in temper; I would not be mad!*

For Lear, as for many in psychosis, a partial recovery comes through sleep, but even sleep cannot, ultimately, protect him.

Timon's character also seems an astute portrait of manic depression. He spends money recklessly until he is bankrupt; his sociability and speediness are excessive; his connectivity extreme: he is impulsive in generosity and hyperbolic in describing it.

> *Methinks, I could deal kingdoms to my friends,*
> *And ne'er be weary.*

His judgement is poor – 'Unwisely, not ignobly, have I given' – and, equally unwisely, he gives himself false consolation, believing 'I am wealthy in my friends.' Not so. As they disperse like mist in sunshine, he falls into an isolated and angry depression.

And then there's Cleopatra, queen of the mood-swingers. One of Shakespeare's later plays, *Antony and Cleopatra* evidences his

ongoing fascination with mercuriality. Cleopatra is volatile, contra-
dictory, emotionally vast, and her language loves extremes: 'Eternity
was in our lips and eyes.' She is given to violence and finally commits
suicide in flaming language:

> *I am fire and air; my other elements*
> *I give to baser life.*

It is impossible not to see in Cleopatra the temperament of manic
depression, but in *The Winter's Tale* Shakespeare locates bipolarity
not in a character but in the play itself, with its first half Tragedy
and second Comedy, hinged on the central character of Autolycus
as every winter's tale is hinged at the door of January, Janus the
two-headed, and as theatre itself is symbolized by two faces, one
tragic, one comic.

And I, meanwhile, was also at the hinge of the year, my mind
ajar in January.

PART FOUR:
TILL THE LIGHT

It was in the dark days of January that I became feverish to write the poetry of this madness. I felt a ferocious need to transmute the pain, to translate the fury and glory from inside to outside.

On the first and maddest night of this episode, Mercury had got the upper hand and had recklessly sent me mad. I had begged not to be sent incurably mad. He looked hell-bent on ignoring my plea, so I had pinioned him to the ground with drugs.

One night, half asleep, I dreamt of a woman saying:

– It's the pylons, Jay.

And I understood the metaphorical truth of that image. The electrical currents in my brain which should be flowing had shorted, the neuro-transmitters (the chemical messengers) had gone berserk and an electrical fire was almost out of control. Almost. The antipsychotics and mood stabilizers were firefighting. I was caught between the wisdom of sanity and the beguiling compulsion of madness. The leaflet with the pills I was taking said they 'correct the functioning of the neurotransmitters'. *Take that, Mercury.* But he prowled, only half corrected, through my nights and days, making each one last a year. He cast spells of furious intensity, such messages from my memories that I was shocked into childhood. I was all the ages of my life, in one breathless present.

I let my doctor persuade me to take slightly higher doses, but the medication muffled me. At best, I felt like an amiable sheep: I could eat grass and shit by the fence, but without emotion or mindedness, simply as a set of biological compulsions. My emotions seemed to thud against a blanketed wall; they could barely move beyond middle C. At worst, I felt straitjacketed on the inside, a trapped animal, psyche snared.

I was bargaining hard with Mercury. Give me metaphor, and I'll let you run wild in my mind. But if you continue to make me lose my mind – and your job in myth was to find Psyche, not to lose her – I will drag you down to earth with drugs. So behave a bit better, Mercury, just a bit, or be damned with drugs, for I have to find a softer landing back to Plynlimon, Powys, happiest county in Britain, of which I am not a shining example.

Then Mercury offered truce terms to psychiatry in turn. Now *he* was plea-bargaining:

– Keep the doses low and I'll give you poems.

Deal.

A game of forfeit, played for poems.

Always dangerous, though, to deal with Mercury, the god unbound, who keeps no promises, honours no bargains and pays no bills. But, in this fragile peace accord, I wrote poems over the course of three weeks in January, in the rift of time, the hours between three in the morning when I woke and the first light at eight o'clock and the stirrings of the ordinary sounds of the traffic of life in my little town, as the first car drives past.

Meanwhile, a friend of mine, a retired psychiatrist, had returned to my town after some weeks away. She had heard that I was ill and came to see me. Andy is eccentric to the point of social concavity.

She is wild, chaotic and deeply kind. She's the sort of person there is no 'sort' for. Some years back, following a conversation with a Labour local councillor over inadequate housing for elderly people, she bought a plot of land so the council could build sheltered housing. But the opening ceremony was commandeered by a Tory bigwig, and she was so disgusted by his politics that she presented him with a cake she'd made herself, out of cow shit. Doctor, farmer, mother, activist, ruder than giant hogweed at the Chelsea Flower Show, Andy brought a clarity and strength I needed.

— I don't want to go mad, I said, imploring.

— They all say that, she answered. Everyone with manic depression in crisis.

— And I don't want to commit suicide, I said, naming the stalking fear.

— They all say that, she replied.

— And I want to bring something back.

— They all say that, too.

— So I'm quite normal for mad?

She gave me a look more grimace than grin.

My psyche was on a dangerous journey, but a further reach of the human mind comes within one's grasp in those extra octaves, something exquisite and oddly impersonal. It is accented by one's individual nature, yes, but still seems to touch something beyond, a cry for the divine. I had to write poetry not in spite of madness but because of it, knowing something mythic is here in the numinous human mind.

A friend, with perfect timing, said to me at this point:

— Write. Right now. Don't lose these thoughts, this experience.

The composer Sally Beamish, who used to be a viola player, tells the story of how she began composing after her house was burgled and thieves stole her precious viola. She turned to composing in consolation. I felt forced to poetry when madness stole my prose.

I do not write poetry; or, rather, I had never done so. Now there was no question in my mind that I had to and that I could write nothing except poetry. I normally never write at night but now I could write only in darkness. Normally, I cannot write without a decent amount of sleep but now I was jolted awake at three in the morning, after a bare three hours' sleep. And so, with the poet Francis Thompson, 'I laughed in the morning's eyes.'

In the daytimes I became nothing, I did nothing, had no mattering and was dissolved. At night, though, for three weeks between January 5th and January 25th, I became myself. I wrote through everything, including what would turn out to be the single most dangerous night: January 18th. Why am I writing the dates? Usually, I am cavalier about the precise dates of things because that seems the least important part of any description. In this madness, though, dates seemed to be something to hold on to, as if they belonged, with strict rationality and housework, to the clarity of sanity and sense which I clung to in my daylight mind.

Awake at night, though, stalking poems, a poacher in paradise, I was searching in the fields of madness for the jawbones of the gods.

I didn't really care if these poems were good or bad; if medicine cures, it is irrelevant whether it tastes bitter or sweet. I had to write without censoring myself, to curl mania around and bring it home safe; to make a path of honest words, to write the truths which save the psyche, not because the words would be perfect but because they would be present and pure. In the darkness of night and illness, I could riddle the stars for their sparks.

It seems there is a strong relationship between suffering and poetry. Literary critic Leon Edel once said: 'Out of world-sadness, out of tristimania, immortal and durable things are brought into being.' Shelley was to write:

> *Most wretched men*
> *Are cradled into poetry by wrong,*
> *They learn in suffering what they teach in song.*

Orpheus, legendary poet, takes Eurydice's hand to draw her out of the underworld, and when he looks back, and loses her, Pluto tells him: 'Your wife is payment for your poems.' Poets pay a devastating price in the coin of suffering, and when Anne Sexton writes, 'Poetry led me by the hand out of madness,' it sounds curative but it is also possible to see in it a warning. Following Orpheus but stumbling like Eurydice, Sexton is one of so many poets to have committed suicide.

If there is no doubting the relationship between the ability to suffer and the need to write poetry, so there is also no doubting the way in which poetry eases suffering. Cowper wrote that, in states of distress, 'I find writing, especially poetry, my best remedy.' In the nineteenth century, people in mental asylums were encouraged to write poetry, with positive results. Les Murray wrote: 'I'd disapproved of using poetry as personal therapy, but the Black Dog taught me better. Get sick enough, and you'll use any remedy you've got.' Recollecting the schoolteachers who introduced him to poetry, Murray calls it 'an art form they may have guessed might save me, even as my unconscious aptitude for it might have caused my miseries'. Poetry is both cause and cure.

In Dante's time, books were bought in apothecary shops; litera-ture sold as medicine. (Dante himself became a pharmacist, needing to be a member of a guild in order to take public office.) There is a deeper metaphor at work here – that the apothecary of language can heal first the writer and then the reader.

The links are there in myth, for Apollo is god of poetry and medicine and Orpheus is the renowned hero of poetry who is like-wise associated with healing, while his lyre has the power to vanquish melancholy. So powerful was his art that he charmed animals and birds – even stones – but he was killed by those unable to appreciate his art. The vicious maenads first attacked him with sticks and stones, but this failed because the rocks and branches loved him so much they refused to hit him. So the enraged women tore him to pieces. Orpheus is gone but he leaves traces – his song was taken up by trees, rocks and rivers, as if he had left his gift of healing immanent in the care of the natural world.

To heal is to make whole, and when the mind is broken poetry can work towards healing it, uniting it with itself and reconnecting it with the world. Art comprehends us – it is through language that we are understood – and poetry, above all, steps into the heart and saturates it with understanding. Whenever I read poetry which has this kind of knowledge, I know that I am known. I am seen. I am not alone. How to understand a text is a matter of pedagogy. How to be understood by a text is a matter of healing. In the awful loneli-nesses of depression and the bleak, mind-swept realms of madness, poetry comes kind to hand, offering to unpuzzle silence.

When the psyche is ill, the world can seem inchoate and unword-able, but poetry, shaping words, gives form to formlessness; it threads words like beads on a line to lead you up from the underworld.

And when poetry comprehends mania, it can be electrifying: Christopher Smart in 'A Song to David' writes of:

> *Notes from yon exaltations caught,*
> *Unrival'd royalty of thought.*

In medicine I saw the science of pain but in poetry I saw pain's art. Medicine has an anaesthetic relationship to pain – it wants to rid the patient of it. Poetry has an aesthetic relationship to pain – it wants pain to speak. And the illness which seems to want to speak itself more than any other is manic depression. It is itself a storyteller, seeking uninhibited mouths through which to utter. Théophile Gautier wrote of Gérard de Nerval's poem 'Aurélia': 'It has been said of "Aurélia" that it is a poem in which madness tells her own story. It would have been even more accurate to describe it as Reason writing the memoirs of Madness at her dictation.'

In medicine, pain is an enemy, held at lancet-length, and there is a simple ethical quest to overcome it. In poetry, pain is a companion, the wounded-healer needs to hold hurt hard by, a complex of injured-knowing held behind the eyes.

Medicine's science of pain is observant, paying attention to pain's symptoms to make pain obedient to experiment and the laws of chemistry. In poetry's art, pain is impetuous, disobedient; it has a life of its own, lifting off the page, vitally alive, leaving a scent of sea or civet and leaping onwards.

Medicine's science of pain seeks balance and asks for the typical aetiology, searching for patterns of illness and predictable outcomes. Poetry's art of pain eschews the norm, to sniff out the idiomatic. If medicine measures pain, poetry longs for pain's immeasurable echoes.

Medicine tests its hypotheses while poetry would take hypotheses for fireworks. Medicine likes Occam's razor, using the simplest explanation until that is proved insufficient; poetry would use Occam's razor only to slit its wrists.

John Keats – a licensed apothecary – trained unhappily as a doctor when he should have been working as a poet, and suffered depression accordingly: his brother wrote of him that John 'feared that he should never be a poet, and if he was not he would destroy himself'. It is an illustration of what happens when the poet is stifled (or self-stifling), for depression (or manic depression) can be seen as the result of an unanswered calling. Gwyneth Lewis, in her memoir of depression, recounts how it was her resistance to writing poetry that made her ill: 'If you don't do what your poetry wants you to, it will be out to get you. Unwritten poems are a force to be feared.' In a wider sense, those who refuse their vocation may be maddened by it to the point of serious illness. A Yale University study by Paul B. Lieberman and John S. Strauss suggested a trigger for people's manias was the 'enforced pursuit of an activity that was at odds with their own goals and aspirations'. The Gnostic Gospel of Thomas portrays Jesus saying: 'If you bring forth what is within you, what you bring forth will save you. If you do not bring forth what is within you, what you do not bring forth will destroy you.'

In our society, poetry and the arts are the last culturally accepted forms in which shamanism exists and, as we've seen, cultures which have retained their shamanism hold a widespread understanding that shamans who resist their vocation become ill while the practice of that shamanism will be their cure. Perhaps artists who do not practise their vocation risk such psychological crisis that they simply *cannot* work in regular, habituated ways, because the work of the soul is calling and cannot be ignored.

It is a matter of being allowed to become who you truly are, to express your exact self, precisely delineated, each of us our own *logos*, exactly defined, evolved into ever more discriminated a meaning. Mercury is the individuating principle, according to Jung, who helped people (and things) towards their quiddity, their this-ness. Only through individuation – becoming most fully yourself – can you fully enter into a relationship with others. Part of this individuation, in Jung's therapeutic practice, included searching for a patient's purpose and meaning. Logotherapy, according to Viktor Frankl, is the process by which each of us discerns our purpose in life, a self-transcendent meaning which is distinctly ours to follow. Aristotle, meanwhile, wrote of happiness as *eudaimonia*, and the term literally means that one's *daemon*, an essential aspect of one's soul, is 'well pleased', that one is flourishing, doing what one does best and doing it with excellence.

Meanwhile, the contemporary Icarus Project was created to 'navigate the space between brilliance and madness'. Of manic depression, the founders write: 'We see our condition as a dangerous gift to be cultivated and taken care of rather than as a disease or disorder needing to be "cured" or "eliminated".' The project uses myth and metaphor for a manifesto of inspiration, as opposed to regarding madness purely as illness and dysfunction.

Enid Welsford describes the role of the old Irish *fili*, or poet, as being one who was very highly trained in poetry, story, history and law. The *fili* must understand 'the secret language of the poets', which Welsford suggests perhaps refers to a time when 'mastery of metaphor' was not an art but a science, 'the mark of initiation into an esoteric code'. It makes me wonder whether there is an esoteric code within the human mind for the mind's self-description in episodes of madness: otherwise, why do the metaphors cohere?

Hurricanes, cliffs, abyssal depths, oceans and black dogs are such common descriptions of bipolar or unipolar states that it seems there may be a kind of collective unconscious at work.

In madness, just as in art, the individual human mind reaches out beyond itself, outside its own life towards a larger sense of Life. In ancient Greek understanding, life in its form of *bios* is partial, individual, conscious and personal, existing in time. Life in its form of *zoe*, though, is concerned with the whole, the eternal, the collective, unconscious and archetypal. Zoë Playdon writes: 'This relationship between *bios* and *zoe*, between time and eternity, between the individual and the archetypal, is the central concern of Greek myth.' It is also a central concern of art and, indeed, madness, where *bios* reaches outwards towards *zoe*.

In these days, I was still spending hours playing the piano, because music harmonized me. As someone with a stammer might be able to sing fluently, so, although my days stuttered over quotidian logic, yet my fingers could make music. I poured myself into poetry and piano-playing. If I wasn't doing either, though, I could feel panic rising and the only reliable anti-panic device was counting the days and then the hours before my next appointment with my doctor. *If I can just get through three days, I'll be safe. If I can just hang on four hours, I'll be able to talk to him.* As long as the spaces between appointments were a length of time which I could picture – in practice, three days – then I felt less panicky. I could imagine Today, Tomorrow and The Day After Tomorrow, but that was all. The appointments themselves calmed me, but simply the fact of having a fixed appointment within the visible horizon gave me a lifeline, a rope on the mountain so that I could attach a carabiner. What I didn't know was that I was about to need him urgently for a wholly unforeseeable reason.

I'd written three poems the first morning, three also on the second morning. But that night, my left eye began to hurt to distraction. It had been bloodshot for weeks, beginning exactly when I had started taking the antipsychotic pills. I'd ignored it, thinking it was due to sleeplessness and tobacco smoke; I don't usually smoke and I don't want to smoke, but this had been a steep few weeks on the baccy. Now, though, a month after I'd started taking the antipsychotic, the redness suddenly worsened.

In the worst of crisis. The eye of the storm. Is blood.

Then, on the third poetry day, my sight was clouded as if I were looking through a screen of pearly silk. And it hurt, aching painfully at any alteration of light. I did not know that the eye itself could hurt like this. The lights which had been metaphorically too bright on the inside of my head were now literally too bright on the outside. At first, I tried to blink repeatedly to clear it, and I dug out some sunglasses and sat in the dark, but it got worse quickly. I phoned my doctor.

He was with a patient. When he phoned me back, I was out, but as I was walking home he was driving away from the surgery and saw me on the street. He stopped me and looked at my eye and got me back into the surgery rapidly. He fixed an emergency eye appointment at a hospital. My pupil had stuck to my iris and the pressure was squeezing the optical nerve to screaming point. The optical nerve can be pinched like this until it is severed. I found out later that, if my doctor had not moved so fast, I could have lost the sight of that eye.

A friend took me to the hospital and I had a manic-attack. I felt something of the gravity of eye emergencies, but the giggle-helium was pumping into me and I was overcome by the raucous cartoonishness of the situation. My pupil wouldn't dilate, so I had to lie on a gurney with a purple plastic Marigold glove full of warm water on my eye. 'We'll be here for a while,' my friend said: 'There are nine hundred gloves. I just counted.' Everything was balloons, inflated, ridiculous, gigglesome.

I left the hospital with steroid eye drops which I had to apply every two hours, night and day, which was hard, as the one thing I needed most was sleep and this extra sleepless stress was likely to make my psychosis (*my* psychosis? are it and I now on friendly terms?) worse. But I would have my sight.

Drug companies are under no obligation to publish complete information about side effects; about half of all clinical results are published, and that half is chosen by drug companies. It probably won't amaze you to learn that positive results are roughly twice as likely to be published as negative ones.

Obviously, it would be impossible to prove that it was the anti-psychotic which caused this potential blinding, but my eye had been affected from the day I began taking it and began to recover the day I stopped. This serious potential reaction to the antipsychotic was not published as a possible side effect of the drug, but my doctor reported my case on the Yellow Card Scheme, which is set up to identify adverse drug reactions which might not otherwise be known. What will the company do with that information? Turn a blind eye, I imagine.

Strangely, in this psychological illness of two halves – half manic, half depressed – my body followed suit. It split down the middle. On the right side, I was fine. On the left side, my eye was damaged. It was my left ankle which I'd hurt so badly falling down the rabbit hole. My left shoulder was hurting and I couldn't do cartwheels because of an old injury now troubling me again. Ankles and shoulders are joints and joining points – the Trickster body parts – and were playing up. Then the glands on the left side of my body began swelling. Ear, neck, armpit. But all their opposite numbers on the right side were absolutely fine; just the ones on the left had gone wayward. Of the brain's two hemispheres, the left is more given to logic and rationality: the right is more gifted at insight, music, metaphor and jokes. It was as if the left side of my body were weirdly chiming in, a mind-body rhyme of brokenness.

If the pupil of my eye was learning somatically, what exactly could I see? This blindedness coinciding with poetry was like a somatic performance of insight: the eye of the mind can see further and more deeply than literal sight can reach. I could write only by night, when darkness made things visible. In gorgeous spiralling hallucinations, I had been seeing things that didn't exist, but now I could not see things which did.

It was completely out of the question to drive. I felt an odd sense of relief that I had no choice but to stay in the underworld, the dark night of the subconscious. The trappings and harnesses of the dutiful everyday were lifted from me. I was out of the traces, racing the dark for its sight.

I was offered a replacement antipsychotic. I didn't take it. I wanted to stay mad for the poetry I could feel in my fingers. It was a precise parallel to how I have always treated altitude: when I've climbed mountains, I have always been sensible about climbing risks but jeopardized my safety when it comes to altitude sickness. I've never turned back, I've been willing to take the pain and the danger for the views, the summit, the angle of exaltation at the heights.

Mountains were calling me in all ways. I was reckless with the psyche's highs, crying for sky. I wanted to climb Cader Idris again, because it's the closest mountain to where I live. If you spend the night on Cader, they say, you will end up either mad, dead or a poet, and I was poem-stained and maddened enough already, my mind a high-wire, live firework.

I had, much earlier, cancelled all work plans for the foreseeable future: except one. The Royal Shakespeare Company was in rehearsal for *As You Like It*, and they wanted me to talk to the cast about wildness and the Forest of Arden, and to write a programme note on the play. The Otherworld. I didn't need to cancel that because I already was in the Forest of Arden, and with the depression of Jaques and the irritable mania of Touchstone to boot.

But the big work event which I could not cancel was the publication of *Kith*, scheduled for March, and looming, tense, monstrous and terrifying to me. I hadn't lacked confidence in the process of writing, and both my agent and editor loved the book, but its publication felt utterly beyond me. It would demand press interviews, BBC broadcasts, as well as readings and talks at literature festivals. I felt like a kayaker at sea in a night fog seeing the hull of an enormous freighter set on an inexorable course towards me. I would far preferred to have been able to slink off into ornamental hermitude for a few months, but I felt I owed it to my work to do the media rounds which publication required, though the idea made me shaky and tearful. My doctor, though, was telling me over and over again that I should have no pressures at all and urged me to postpone it.

I was at that point waking sharply every hour, my dreams fouled with nightmare churning up from psyche's mud, and these nightmares were so bad I dreaded going to bed. Suicide was knocking at the door. At this point in my notebook, it says: 'so hard to manage journey back from London then crashed at home – ways to do it?' *It* being suicide. Thinking about that made me go back to Mercury, furious, white-lipped, intense. Give me poems and let me come back *safe*: that was the deal. Psychopomp, guide of souls, guide me back. As if.

My notebook, in mid-January, records: 'Desperate: Sat day, Sat night, Sun night, Mon day, Mon night.' Something terrible was on the way and my heart was tumbling, sometimes beating so erratically that I was short of breath.

What kind of drunk you are sometimes seems in the lap of the gods. Some people are violent drunks; some are spiteful, aggressive or argumentative. Some are grandiose, some giggly, some maudlin, weepy or affectionate. What kind of manic you are also feels down to the luck of the draw. I felt lucky because, although I was more irritable than I would be normally, it was seldom directed at others. I don't get aggressive or paranoid. Even though I'd been hallucinating, I wasn't delusional: a distinction which may be hard to understand from the point of view of someone who has not experienced it. To explain: even when I could 'see' – in that dreamlike trance – a hallucination, I knew, rationally, that it was not there. It felt more like seeing my dreams and my metaphors. This isn't to say that my mind was controlled: it wasn't. I felt like a goose flying dangerously out of the V-shape of the skein, frantically pecking at the air with my beak and clutching wings, grabbing at clear sky with my goose feet, flapping, ugly and panicky.

I also feel lucky with manic depression in that I have years at a stretch without depression's dreaded tap on the shoulder. I've only had two steep episodes of hypomania in my life, rather than the constant cycling of highs and lows which many people experience. But suicide has harried me in my worst times. In one depression in my twenties I stood around at the gates of a mental hospital, desperately trying to walk in, but I couldn't because I didn't feel I mattered enough. Then I crossed and re-crossed the road without looking, hoping I'd get hit by a car and have to be admitted to some kind of hospital, at least. Cars beeped and swerved, and one driver yelled abuse at me, which brought me back to at least a fraction of my senses.

On the cover of the first of my notebooks from this current episode, I'd drawn an exploding star. On the next, I'd drawn a feather, for both flight and writing. On the third, I drew a mountain with the sharp, jagged heights of an Alpine silhouette.

During this stage of my madness, I lived in the mountains of the mind, the kind which Gerard Manley Hopkins knew, his 'cliffs of fall'. By choice, I'd spent the previous ten days in the death zone. I did it so that I could write the essence of the poems, so I could bring something back out of all these awful months, something of a record. But now, just as with physical climbing, the issue was how to get down safely, how to get off the mountain without having to be helicoptered off, without coming down in a body-bag. *More accidents happen on the way down*, I reminded myself over and over, and made myself start taking the replacement antipsychotic.

I took the first pill at four thirty in the afternoon one day and fell asleep from five thirty to seven thirty and then slept from eleven until six in the morning. A total of nine sweet hours: more than I had slept in months. When I woke, I felt like crying for Hopkins and John Clare, for Kit Smart and Coleridge – and all the unknown people who have walked this curly cliff-edge living too early in history for this kind of help. And I realized just how suicidal I had felt when I realized that the feeling had ebbed. (For the moment.) In the twelve hours after that first pill, I felt I'd climbed down at least to an altitude where there was enough oxygen, and I could see how close I had been. Andy said later that she had been very concerned at that point because, she said, I didn't *sound* right. Long ago, I read that a crucial suicide clue is the voice: the time to worry seriously is when someone is speaking in an utterly flat tone, a hollow monotone without intonation. That is where I'd been.

More accidents happen on the way down, I repeated. In the literal mountains, this is because climbers are tired and, after the fierce focus on getting to the summit, their attention is dispersed. Take your eye off the target and your feet slip; the mind, without its edge of ambition, is a blunted blade, its judgement unsharpened. More accidents may happen on the way down, too, I thought, in the mountains of the mind. It was possibly my physical knowledge of mountains that prepared me at some level for what was coming.

Postponing a book's publication, at barely two months' notice, is not a small thing for a publisher. The knock-on effects can be difficult and tedious, unexpected and awkward, all together. But I realized I had to ask. I called my editor and my agent and explained quite how ill I was. They rallied round me with a speed, care and emotional intelligence I'll always be grateful for. They made me feel that publication was as easy to reschedule as a pint down the pub. (It wasn't.) They gave me the chance to choose a revised publication date without speed or pressure, and more than anything they gave me a sense of care – even love.

The publication date was put back, removing for a while my fear. But something else was coming: I felt dread, a sense of constant emergency. I'd reverted to waking at 3 a.m. and, in this frozen January, those night hours were still and quiet enough to hear the gods.

I live in a small town in the hills and in the summers I like walking, running, swimming, biking and horse riding. In the winters, I like tobogganing as well and, the height of my pleasure, skating on frozen lakes. In this illness, I was desperate to be outside: mania charges me with the electricity of intense vigour which seeks to be discharged, to be spent. But this winter's weather prohibited everything. It was too icy to go running or even walking, let alone horse riding, as the stones and rocks were like wet glass and I'd nearly fallen badly twice and I didn't want to risk hurting my ankle again. There was ice everywhere but, really disappointingly, the ice on the lakes was not thick enough to skate on. There had been a slight snowfall, but not enough to toboggan. I was pacing like a wild cat, agitated, despairing, caged.

If I felt trapped physically with that unusual combination of weather factors, I also felt caged in time, in one trapped now. As if in one terrible tripping of the switches, there had been a massive signal failure in my brain and all the depressions I'd ever had were now shunted together like train carriages in a derailment, each previously separate carriage shoved into one compacted whole, a gargoyle of twisted metal.

I spoke to several friends about suicide and one said she believed people have a choice and no one should try to stop someone who wants to do it. I felt juddered, shaken into unsafety by this, for while I agree that if someone in their right mind (perhaps towards the end of life, with an incurable disease) chooses to walk out into the snow with a fistful of pills and a crate of champagne, that is their right, but I would want to be stopped by any means necessary.

My notebook at this point is littered with the word 'suicide', and the statistics compilers, a benevolent force of cautious, serious understanding, seemed oddly helpful. Knowing that one in five people in this state commit suicide is sobering. Added to this, writing is a profession with a high suicide risk. *Think on't*, the facts seemed to say. Tread very, very carefully. I'd attempted (if that's the word) suicide when I was twenty, in a cack-handed, lackadaisical, be-drunken despair, swallowing a bottle of paracetamol in front of my boyfriend, who then shoved a toothbrush down my throat till I spewed. Yuck: the vile indignity of the young drunk. I remember a nurse and a liver-function test.

Meanwhile, my friends were openly talking about hospitalization. I was frightened to talk about it with my doctor, because I dreaded bringing on myself the fearful necessity of dealing with unknown people (staff and patients) and I was frightened of being beyond his care, out of his hands. He said later that he thought hospitalization would make me worse, and that the other patients, in particular, would affect me badly. I'm sure he was right about that: at one point in this episode, I met a friend of a friend in the local café who tried to talk to me about her madness in a psychiatric hospital. Her psyche played chords which set up resonances in mine, and in that comprehended cacophony I felt pure panic. I had to get up and leave, mid-conversation.

Being hospitalized, said my doctor, might mean being sent a long way away from home, away from my friends. He was, I could see, trying hard to assess just how suicidal I was. This is a merciless place for a doctor to be. If they don't get a patient hospitalized – sectioned, if necessary – and then a patient talking suicide actually goes and does it, there would be serious questions for a doctor to answer: should have – could have – done different. I think it would have been far easier for him to get me into hospital, but I felt he was putting my need above his and was therefore holding a heavy responsibility, and, since I'd refused to go back to the psychiatrist, he was, in terms of the medical system, holding this responsibility alone.

The trouble with trying to assess whether someone is suicidal is that sometimes they themselves do not know. I couldn't judge whether or not I would try it. My assessment was poor on every count. What I could do, though, was be totally frank about it, day by day. In this state of mind, honesty feels life-saving and lies are killing machines. On the one hand it feels imperative not to cry wolf, even by accident, and on the other it feels utterly necessary never to understate how suicidal I was, because my safety depended on that.

In my mind, I was on a bare mountain, in winter. The weather was against me and my last shred of good judgement was to acknowledge that my judgement was very poor and that I needed to listen to people whose judgement I had previously known to be good. My fail-safe lifeline on this mountain was the rope which attached me to my doctor, like the lead climber, leading, *docens*, as a good doctor can. Without that rope, I would fall, possibly fatally.

And then the avalanche.

There was a sudden, enormously heavy snowfall on Friday 18th January. I had an appointment booked with my doctor for five. In the morning, feeling the snow to be a reprieve from my indoor jail, I gathered up my warmest gear and my sledge and went tobogganing in the hills with a friend. The dread was with me but it is hard not to feel at least a little health and invigoration sledging in deep snow. All day, the snow was piling in cornices and banks, and in the afternoon I tobogganed home, as the roads were perfect sledge-runs and empty of cars. Even a snow plough needed a snow plough ahead of it, and as the snow was falling so thickly it was impossible to keep the roads clear. Nothing could move on the roads, nothing. Except a sledge.

I got home to find several messages from the surgery saying they had to close early because of the snow, and that my doctor had been trying to rearrange an appointment with me for earlier in the day. But by the time I'd picked up the messages, he had left. The soonest appointment I could make with him would be for the following Tuesday.

The metaphoric world is clandestine much of the time but on occasion it takes on the form of reality. The mythic werewolf or werejaguar crosses between realities; partly living in the human world, partly in the world of wolf or jaguar. Now, metaphor itself was shapeshifting into a kind of were-reality, if you will, but one so true I could almost mistake it for the real thing. I was on a mountain in deep snow and an avalanche had swept the lead climber away from me, out of sight, beyond hearing. There was an inward and near-fatal avalanche in my mind. Alone, with the accumulated dread of the last few days coursing through me, I felt pure panic shooting through my veins. The pulse in my head became unbearable. The inexorable drumming had begun again.

I had a choice. I could do the sensible thing on a mountain: stay calm, hunker down, scoop out a basic snow shelter, wait it out until I could find my lead climber again, and then, with clear skies and roped on, I would be safe. That was what the voice of reason would have said. But my reason had deserted me and other voices called, which I could hear. Not as some people literally hear voices but more like hearing the echoes of a dream. Instead of being sad, stuck and forced to wait out these dreadful days, I could move – in fact, I *had* to move, to go somewhere, somehow, my own way, and unharnessed if necessary. The allure lay that way.

So I did the worst thing you can do on a sheer rock face in heavy snow: I panicked. I got drunk and I didn't take that evening's medication – the equivalent of taking off the carabiner and safety harness and failing to use the safety rope. And then I tried a tricky traverse, alone.

Into suicide, black against the snow.

A death flit, a traverse at night on a bare, raw mountain, edged like a razor, like a knife, like scissor-points, like the blade of a Stanley knife. I went round the house, gathering them all up. And then I began this dangerous essay.

None of the scissors were sharp enough. I have never sharpened my kitchen knives. But the Stanley knife, pressed into my wrist, felt as if it could do the job. A knife must move to make cuts; it must slice. It is a horribly brutal sight to see a blade against human skin, and then I realized that, no matter what else, I didn't have the necessary violence.

I phoned the Samaritans. They were engaged. In a kind of gallows humour, I felt like laughing at this bitter joke. *Unbefuckinglievable.* Now. This night. When all my life was shrunk to a crucible, boiled down to pure, toxic pain: now. The Samaritans Are Engaged.

Suddenly, I heard a commotion downstairs in the kitchen. I went to see what it was, still holding the Stanley knife in my hand. One of my cats had killed a bird, a treecreeper, a very shy woodland bird and not one you'd ever normally see in town, but I suppose this snow had made it as desperate in its way as I was in mine. It jolted me: the violence of the cat's claws had raked cruel gouges of razor marks all down the bird's back. I felt sick and faint, reeling into real reality. This is Knife. This is Killing. This is Violence. This is Death, for real. It was as if this bird played the part of a sacrifice: its death shocked me out of my own.

I dropped the knife in the kitchen and, too shaken to do anything else, shut the cat into the kitchen with its kill. And the knife. And the alcohol.

And then I wished so keenly to be able to ring 999 and ask for an ambulance, to admit myself anywhere but here, this death-darkened house, to go into any kind of hospitality. I needed other voices, more sensible than mine, voices which were wise and kind, which I could tune into.

I called Andy.

– Don't do anything stupid, she said bluntly: no ambulance would be able to get to you tonight.

I was crying and found it hard to speak but, as before, I needed to listen more than to talk.

– Have you taken your medication?

– No.

– Why not?

– I want to die.

– You can't really want to kill yourself or you wouldn't have phoned me.

(I can't fault the logic.)

– I want to die. And I don't. I'm trying not to.

– Go to bed: nothing terrible can happen if you go to bed. Make yourself a cup of tea and go to bed.

– I don't drink tea this late in the day. If I do, I won't sleep.

An absurdist playwright has been let loose in our dialogue. I had phoned her at very midnight, hysterically suicidal, and now I was explaining that I'm very sensitive to caffeine and a diddly cup of tea would keep me awake all night. Mind on parallel lines: the ordinary and the opera. But, somehow, hearing these words coming out of my mouth, no matter how bizarre under the circumstances, was like a first step towards normal. 'Often, people want both to live and to die; ambivalence saturates the suicidal act,' writes Kay Redfield Jamison in *Night Falls Fast*.

– Anyway, I can't get to the kitchen.

– Why not?

– There's a dead bird in there.

(Pause.)

– So?

– I'm frightened of dead birds.

(Exasperated pause.)

– Look, can you take the pills, and stay on the phone while you get into bed?

– I don't know.

– What don't you know?

(Again, absurdity strikes: maybe she thought I didn't know if I could make myself take the medication, or be able to go to bed. Maybe she thought I'd walk out into the snow.)

– *What* don't you know? she asked again.

– I don't know if the phone cord is long enough to reach into my bedroom.

It's heavenly-daft, looking back on that conversation from a very different place, but it surprises me still how the mind, when mad, can hold in the same moment ideas of terrible heft and also the desultory trivia of caffeine sensitivity and length of phone cords.

The phone line did stretch, and I did take the pills, in bed.

– Stay there, Andy said. I can't get to you till it's light.

Even her four-wheel drive hadn't been able to get up the hill to her house, so she'd have to wait till morning, walk to her vehicle, then drive down to me.

– Just stay in bed. I'll be there at eight.

She was. Thank all the gods. She was tactful, slow, sensitive. This seriously worried me: she is robust with the robust, kind to those off-kilter, but when she's this gentle, you know two things: one is that you're very ill and the other is that you're in good hands.

She called the duty psychiatrist to discuss what to do, and she spoke to me very carefully.

– Do you *want* to end up in hospital?

– Actually, at the moment, yes.

– I meant it as a rhetorical question.

– I wouldn't mind.

– What I mean is you're in danger of being sectioned if you carry on like this much longer.

– Yup.

I could see her point.

She drove me to stay with friends who live an hour away. Getting away completely from the place where you've been thinking about suicide is important, Andy said. I knew I would feel safe with these friends. More specifically, I knew that I wouldn't commit suicide in someone else's house because a feeling of politeness would stop me. Does this, too, seem absurd? The incongruence of an etiquette of suicide? It is very rude to kill yourself in someone else's house. It really is the height of bad manners to leave a bloodstained corpse in someone else's bathroom. And just because I didn't matter didn't mean that other people didn't either. So if I was in someone else's house, I'd be safe.

We got to the lane they live on, high in the Welsh hills, but I couldn't find their house, although I'd been there dozens of times. In this snow, everything was becoming everything else, there were no perspectives and I couldn't get my bearings. It mirrored my state of mind, and I'd lost my way; all my ways. The lane petered out into a bank of snow and it was clear we had gone past their house, so we turned round. I felt panicky and rolled a cigarette, as if, by seeing myself manage something actual and practical with my hands, my brain might take the cue and follow suit. It didn't. Andy asked a guy walking nearby, and the problem was solved: we were, in fact, all but opposite their house, but the world had become unrecognizable to me – except as a reflection of my inner state: a white-out of the mind.

These details: the losing, the panic, the finding, the titchy stitches of someone's minute doings – why am I describing them here? Because – and I know I'm not alone in this – when someone's psyche has gone awry, they 'read' the world symbolically, particularly in its precise relation to their mind at that point. The world sucks intensity into it. Things do not seem accidental or incidental but loaded with meaning; the inner theatre is staged outside oneself.

The four-wheel drive would not make it up the steep path to my friends' house and the sky was heavy with an imminent fresh snowfall. Andy urgently needed to turn round and get home. I started walking. A hundred yards. Alone. I felt as if I were floundering in miles of Arctic ice, walking to the North Pole. As if two minutes were two months to a bipolar explorer. In moments like this, I can understand something of catatonia: the psyche staggers before the immensity of the moment, the freighted, frightening boulder of everything. Its import, heft and weight are overwhelming.

And then I saw one of my friends at the top of the track and he came down towards me and did the simplest and sweetest thing: he just took my hand in his, like a tug boat to a sinking vessel, and pulled me up through the snow to the house.

All through the day, I had phone calls from friends, widely scattered round the country but tightly connected to each other now. They all said the same thing in almost the same words. It seemed like an urgent council-meet had been called so that they would all be repeating to me the one wisest message: Take the medication or you will be hospitalized. If you're sectioned, you'll lose a lot of autonomy, you'll be out of your doctor's care and in the hands of strangers, and you'll be miles away from us all (though one friend said if I was hospitalized, she would simply move in with me for the duration, at which point utter gratitude welled up in me). Hospital. I think I am already there, I said. The words 'hospital' and 'hospitality' are related, and my friends gave me both.

What did they do that was so healing? They gave me a room which was small and simple: this helped, because there was almost nothing in it that would speak itself or intrude. It was quiet and warm and I felt utterly safe, safe as an animal in its nest. They filled the room with thick, soft duvets and cats and pillows and hot-water bottles. I could sleep a little. They cooked for me and I could eat a tiny bit. Sometimes I wanted to talk endlessly, and they listened, and sometimes I couldn't speak and they didn't mind me, and sometimes I wanted to listen and they were sage and kind – and funny. And they gave me jobs to do, simple, physical jobs which I could do with someone else, like clearing snow off the path, washing up, cleaning the floors, and clearing more snow. I thought fondly of the pejorative term 'basket-case', suddenly seeing how wise it is to give ill people a simple, repetitive physical task: weaving a basket would be something I could do. Anything physical, anything practical. Because seeing myself as useful (no matter in how small a way) was like a Way Back to my normality. Seeing myself creating something, even just a clean plate, was like seeing the chance of creating wellness. Clearing snow made me see the possibility of clearing my mind. It opened a path to my own future.

I concentrated on what my friends were saying, I listened and I took the pills. Three days later, one of my friends drove me home so I could get to an appointment with my doctor. As soon as I saw him, the weekend's whole sorry story fell out of my mouth: the snow, an avalanche to me, the cancelled appointment, my panic, getting drunk, skipping pills, getting suicidal, Andy, everything.

He was, he said, really sorry about the cancelled appointment. I hated what could feel like the narrative of manipulation: if an appointment is cancelled, I will want to kill myself. Nothing in all the degrees of my despair was intended manipulatively, but the narrative, the blunt cause-and-effect, would possibly make someone feel guilty. It would be stupid, unfair and horribly unjust.

Sometimes it is the simplest of phrases which express the truth the best, the monosyllables of deepest feeling. *I need you*, I said, choked, and I realized I had never in my life said those words to anyone. Ever. I needed him like nothing and no one in my life. I had no idea need could be like this. Craven, absolute, stricken need. I needed the force field of safety he created for me. I needed his kindness, the purest ingredient in medication; I needed the way he listened and let me reach him and, likewise, I needed the way he could speak across the gulf of madness towards where my psyche was, wherever it was.

And that was when I saw his wings.

They were long and slender, slate-grey, folded like a swallow's wings, every feather tuned to the currents of the air, ready but waiting, patient, calm and thoughtful. I didn't tell him at the time; I thought he would find it disconcerting.

After that suicide night, I felt as if I was walking into the world again, myself the same and yet different. A subterranean transformation had occurred, as if I had been to my underworld and returned. I had gazed, hypnotized, at death and then bent my sights upwards to life, trying not to look back. In the absence of my own mind, wisdom, strength or wellness, my friends had given me theirs, as if we were all members of Friendly Societies of emotional assurance, each insuring each other against ruin. In this long episode, they had dug deep and found the golden coins. If mania contains a gift for giving, depression needs to practise the gift of receiving, and I had to receive all that was gentle, kind and good which surrounded me.

But if madness can elicit extraordinary protection, it can also, worryingly, provoke a mad cousin. The day I got back home, a friend asked me to supper. She'd heard about my having been suicidal, but we didn't talk about it. She was angry with her partner, so angry that she was screaming and crying, but she was not directing it at him. Purple with rage, she screamed about him, but to me, inches from my face. I was as fragile as I've ever been in my life; fragile as the thinnest glass of an eighteenth-century casement; one breath would shatter it, the echo of one blackbird too close would crack it.

'*You're* suicidal? I want to slit my wrists every *day*,' was the last thing I remember her shouting in fury. I didn't doubt how much pain she was in: I felt sorry that she was so unhappy. But I felt mauled, as if suicidality were suddenly a contest, a rivalry of misery: competitive pain. I felt as if I'd stepped into a mad, dark fairy tale, gargoyles in the castle dungeons, all beak and wings, hunched and ugly, spouting rainwater, both of us imprisoned with sponges of purple fungus oozing in the corners, slugs sickened and self-eviscerating in the gutters.

I had been ill, now, for three months. Returning from the shock of that suicide night took another month. By about mid-February, I could feel shoots of recovery. I hadn't been able to read, because I could not concentrate and words on a page had been like camera images in an old-fashioned darkroom; they slid off the page in a swirl of black ink. Nothing spoke to me unless it precisely comprehended my state of mind, though, if that happened, it felt profoundly healing and I could pay attention. The first book I could read was

Richard Holmes's biography of Coleridge, and my heart went out to Coleridge as if I knew him. If he wasn't writing, walking or with people, he said, 'my feelings drive me almost to agony and madness.'

I could sleep more and eat more come springtime, but I was as weak as a kitten. I lived these weeks in the forest of the mind, at its best the Forest of Arden. All around me were daffodils. I was surrounded by yellowness, the open-hearted, arms-outstretched loveliness of them. And there was no reproach in them. The common life of everything struck me anew this spring, the glow at the heart of it all, the empathic capability of the mind to shapeshift through imagination and a kind of love into any living thing, everyone a Jaques transforming themselves into a stag.

But I was frightened of the depression which almost always follows mixed-state hypomania, depression as simple and horrible as turgid nothingness. I knew that spring can be a difficult time for the damaged mind, precisely because it sharpens the distinction between the lithe, flexing vitality of a rising sun in a young year with the pitiful dredge of the sinking psyche.

Edging out of madness, now, I felt shell-shocked. What *happened* to my *mind*? I remember asking my doctor once. It was like coming to, regaining consciousness in hospital after a serious accident and realizing that something terrible must have happened but having no continuous memory of it. Yes, I had scraps of memory, and those were intensely vivid. Yes, I had written notes to myself over the months, a guard-word of thoughts, to snatch these tatters of time. But I had the bewildering feeling that the last time I looked around me it was November and now it was spring, and every day in that period had been crazy firefighting, not to be mad, not to commit suicide.

This was when my gratitude to my doctor overwhelmed me. He had been doctor, psychiatrist and counsellor. I'm pretty sure he saved my sight. I am absolutely certain he saved my life. There is no gratitude like it.

And then my days began to stumble. They staggered. They fell. It was the awful, inexorable descent into depression. I couldn't write, could still barely read. I felt physically sick thinking about the looming publication of my book and its publicity demands. I had utterly lost confidence in my own wellness at any future time. I couldn't manage to be away from home and couldn't cope with seeing anyone except my phalanx-friends. I was frightened of not washing and becoming part of the stigmatic stench. The rules of self-care became an almost religious duty: to shower, to brush my hair, to wear clean clothes every day. I made to-do lists, and on one day I wrote out the things I was aiming for:

– Put bins out
– Do laundry
– Don't kill myself
– Buy cat food

I had to stop counting the long list of things I couldn't do and start instead with the short list of what I could. I offered myself as a general factotum to my friends. *Just give me a job, a simple job, a physical one.* So I weeded allotments, cleaned gutters, washed up, planted things. A ladder, a scoop and a blocked drainpipe, a wheelbarrow and a pile of earth to move. That kind of thing. Mainly, I tried to stay out of bed and not drink alcohol.

Days turned into weeks which turned into months of utter depression. If my mind had been over-connected and dendritic when I was hypomanic, now it was disconnected from everything. I was back in the 'real' world, out of the faerie world, the woods of midsummer dreams, and into the Court of Athens. And that real world was a painful place to be. I looked around me, aghast at the devastation of days behind me, each new day only an old desolation and nothing in the future but despair. Even God cannot give back the months the locusts took away. Time was a sewer, fetid and blocked underground. I spent a lot of time in the dreamless dirge which passes for sleep; an abnegation of life, a denial of dream, a swimless, flightless annulment. The nothing that will come of nothing.

My doctor gave me antidepressants at the highest dose I'd ever had, nearly five times anything I'd ever taken before. I felt as if my veins were running with water. I dreamt I was crying blood.

'Depression', as a word, does not convey the experience, as William Styron wrote so furiously: 'the word has slithered innocuously through the language like a slug, leaving little trace of its intrinsic malevolence and preventing, by its very insipidity, a general awareness of the horrible intensity of the disease when out of control.' An intensity which Les Murray has called 'shredded mental kelp marinaded in pure pain'. Yes.

Then came the publication of my book, and I was flooded with terrible adrenalin: I was on high alert, in danger. It was an accurate apprehension.

The whole publishing team gave me their utter protection. They stood by me, literally and figuratively, through the upcoming months, giving me support, strength and a sense of safety. Writers I dearly admire, including Philip Pullman, John Berger, Iain McGilchrist; Niall Griffiths and Theodore Zeldin, had loved my book and praised it publicly. It garnered beautiful reviews from people with a literary sensibility and was longlisted for a prestigious literary award in Britain and shortlisted for one in the States. Many readers wrote appreciative letters to me about it.

None of these was enough protection for me in this state. It was the lies which were deadly. One academic used research from my book as if that were her own argument and then presented it as 'evidence' of things my book supposedly lacked. Research references were ignored as if the pages upon pages of notes simply didn't exist. Ideas were misattributed. Metaphor taken literally. So profoundly was my work misrepresented in one newspaper that it had to publish a corrections letter, while its sister paper published such damaging and demonstrably false statements that I wrote to complain. The result? A curt note saying that my remark – challenging a national newspaper on its dishonesty – 'could be taken as defamatory': a veiled threat of libel action – against me.

There is a peculiar, savage, screaming kind of pain in being publicly humiliated. Being lied about in public causes a sense of powerless outrage unlike any other emotion I know. Being bullied, in addition, was beyond my strength.

That was the point at which something in me broke. Utterly and terribly. I felt 'sung', as Indigenous Australians say. Injured, wounded by malevolent, malicious words, poison-tipped to kill the spirit.

A tractate of the Talmud states that to humiliate someone in public is as bad as shedding the blood of another: 'Whoever humiliates another in public is like one who sheds blood,' according to Bava Metzia 58b. In other words, it is one of the most serious sins one can commit, because psychological harm is quite as bad, and often worse, than physical harm.

George Brown, of London University, has devoted himself to studying life events and their impact on the psyche: according to his research, humiliation is a key factor. Severe life events, including many different kinds of loss, can trigger depression, but more precisely they are worst when they include humiliation. Depression, says Richard P. Bentall, is likely to follow humiliation.

'Words! Mere words! . . . Was there anything so real as words?' wrote Oscar Wilde.

There is a particular extra necessity for truth when one is psychologically fragile. 'I can only speak what I perceive to be the truth,' Stephen Fry said once. When Les Murray was asked about depression, he diagnosed a remedy in honesty: 'for self-examination to work, you must tell the exact truth, suppressing nothing.' Poet Gwyneth Lewis maintains: 'Above all, depression is a disease that is concerned with authenticity.'

When you are ill, you have no choice but to be honest; you're stripped bare. Politesse and the elegant chiffon of etiquette are torn to shreds; the suit and tie of manners are crumpled and unwearable. You are naked. People in crisis demand authenticity from others, because inauthentic people have one over you; they may not abuse that power but they have abrogated to themselves the potential to abuse it, and the mad are highly sensitized to the fake or the phoney, which is why people in those episodes have a tendency angrily to reject untruthfulness: because lies create incoherence, which is maddening. Truth is sacred, both to tell the truth, and to have the truth told about you. Truth is also, as Keats knew, beautiful. It reveals, it notices, it listens; it is an active, creative stance in life, and an energizing one. Lies are ugly, silencing, brutal, stupid and deadly. I like the fact that Shakespeare's clown Robert Armin was famous for honesty, and 'honest' was one of the most noted qualities of Shakespeare himself.

Before this whole episode of madness began, I dreamt one night that I was setting off on a long journey to the sea, on a bike, with a horse in a rucksack on my back. Carrying something which could have carried me? Carrying more than I could manage? Or did it refer to my instinct, which was restrained, held in a rucksack from which it was trying to escape but which, if it was allowed its freedom, would be able to carry me? Whatever it meant, I knew one thing now: I would have to play out in daylight the dreams of the night.

PART FIVE:
MIND FLIGHT

I had to walk away. Away from my work, away from my friends, away from my life. Away. I needed to see far horizons again, to realign myself with the realized world of wide mind, long sight and a fineness of things.

For years, I had thought about walking the Camino de Santiago one day, walking right across Spain from the French Pyrenees to the sea on the Galician coast. Suddenly, I knew 'one day' was now.

My preparations were minimal and barely sufficient. I watched the film *The Way*, because I thought I would feel psychologically safer if I had some idea of the path. I tried to reactivate my rocky Spanish. I spent an evening with a friend who had walked the Camino and who gave me priceless advice about what to take. As Little As Possible. This was going to be hard, though, because straight after the month walking the Camino, I was supposed to be flying from Spain to Melbourne, for the Australian publication of my book and a series of media events and festival appearances. I was assuming I'd be well enough by then to manage it. The practical and immediate consequence was that I needed things for Australia, which meant carrying a lot of extra weight.

The Camino de Santiago de Compostela, the full title of the

pilgrim route, means 'The Way of St James of the Field of Stars'. The Camino is over a thousand years old and ends in Santiago or, for those going one step beyond, Finisterre. Opinions differ as to the start of the route, while some say that the pilgrimage necessarily begins where you are: at home. Most often, though, it is begun in St-Jean-Pied-de-Port, in the French Pyrenees, and the journey from there to Santiago is some eight hundred kilometres.

Once I had decided to do it, the wish overtook me and I felt driven by a need at once stubborn and ethereal. I felt like Cyrano de Bergerac's moon voyager, who, captivated by a desire to journey to the moon, encases himself in an iron suit and then throws a magnet moonwards which will pull him up. I would throw the magnet of desire ahead of myself and then be drawn by its force.

It was, under the circumstances, rash, unwise and desperate. But its very desperation spoke: I had no idea what else I could do. I could either linger in that sump of long-term depression, taking more and more pills, my appetite for life failing daily, or I could get my boots on and hurl myself at the road. I was walled in, the room dark with fetid solitude, padlocked by the habit of depression. Pilgrimage might pick the lock; prise open that rusted year.

The body is a self-healing mechanism and undertaking such a long walk would be strong medicine. 'I have two doctors, my left leg and my right,' wrote G. M. Trevelyan. 'When body and mind are out of gear (and those twin parts of me live at such close quarters that the one always catches melancholy from the other), I know that I have only to call in my doctors and I shall be well again.'

I made a list of what I wouldn't take before I made a list of what I would. The first thing I wouldn't take was friends. I felt that for this particular medicine to work I had to go solo. Several friends had offered to walk with me for parts of the route, but I felt that if they came I would attribute my being able to do it to their presence. I needed to know, unequivocally, that I'd done it myself. I needed to show myself that I had won back my own strength, not leant on others. So, no friends. For the same reason I would not take my mobile with me: so that I would have to walk without any voices except my own and that of the path. I was going to do it without tobacco or alcohol because I wanted no cushions or softeners. And, finally, I decided to do it without medication. That last was a unilateral decision and, given the situation I'd been in for the previous nine months, nuts.

One morning, a few days before I was due to leave, I saw two friends of mine on the street; they both seemed cross but, clearly, not with each other. I walked up to them in all innocence and asked who they were so angry with.

— You, Jay, one of them said after a pause.

— And not angry, but concerned.

They thought I was playing with fire, that it was stupid to come off my medication, particularly without talking to my friends, or my doctor, who, between them, had taken custody of my psyche.

— Why haven't you talked to your doctor? they asked.

— Ummm, he's away, I said lamely.

— What would he say if he was here?

— I don't think he'd think it's a good idea.

— And guess what? That's because it *isn't* a good idea. In fact, it's a *terrible* idea and we're *worried* because we *care* about you and we don't want you to end up *suicidal* and *alone* and in another country where none of us can *find* you or even *speak* to you.

(Yes, there were that many italics.)

I backed down, saying I would put the pills in my rucksack, even if I didn't want to put them in my mouth. In the meantime, I prepared the most important thing: an anthology of poems. I asked thirty-three friends to choose a poem for me which they really loved, so that I could read one each day and then pass it on to someone on the path.

Just before the Camino, though, I had a happy promise to fulfil. I have two nephews I adore; the pair of them the apple of my eye. One of them was turning eighteen and I had said I would take him to Paris for his birthday. It was a time of glee, a time out of time. Robust, hilarious, earthy teenage-hood had him in its paws. Part of him was a child still: sweet, affectionate, endearing, playful and giggly. Part of him was a young man: taut, lean and street-wise, his haircut as razor sharp as his wit. He was half kitten, half alley-cat. Those days with him were without question the happiest I had known in eighteen months.

We said our goodbyes in London and I turned back to France, finding my way down to the Pyrenees and realizing by the very first night that this walk, supposed to take about a month, might prove impossible for me to accomplish. The most immediate reason was that I couldn't stop crying. I don't mean that I felt like crying all the time, I mean that I cried, everywhere, continuously. At St-Jean-Pied-de-Port, the evening before leaving, I picked up my *credencial*, the 'pilgrim's passport' which everyone receives at the beginning that is stamped along the way as one stops at hostels or churches. Everyone who walks the Camino is called a pilgrim, which took a little getting used to.

The man in the office wished me *Bon Camino*, and I started crying. I was so lonely, and this was suddenly horrifically hard. I didn't know what to do. So I went into the local church to pray. I don't believe in any kind of god, so I was not praying to anyone or anything. But I was praying, because I simply had no idea what else might work, other than trying to find my strength by imploring it of myself. I prayed for a friend of mine, who was ill. I was carrying a small stone for her, which she had asked me to place on the way. And I prayed for help for myself, to get well by walking.

The first day's walk is thought by many people to be the hardest. It certainly was for me: my rucksack was heavier than anyone else's I met that day because I was carrying all my gear for Australia. I had lost a lot of my accustomed fitness in the months of being so ill. Mainly, though, depression was making every part of me ache. The spirit carries invisible weight, sometimes harder to carry than the body's physical weight. I had come self-laden, heavy of life, lump-loaded and ugly with gravity. This kind of weight is hard to lose. I was also acutely embarrassed about crying all the time, so I was trying to walk without people seeing me, which, given the popularity of the Camino in August, was impossible.

By the time I got to the highest point of the first day, going over Col de Lepoeder, I had a sick headache and was dizzy, faint and confused as to why I was feeling ill. I stopped for hours by a fountain, drinking and resting. Several people tried to persuade me to walk on with them, because they said I looked so ill they thought I shouldn't be alone. Why didn't I say yes to all the offers of help? I didn't really know. It was part of my rigid self-demand to do this walk myself. Being half carried off the mountainside on the first day was not part of my plan. So I ended up walking down alone into the dusk, stumbling, forcing myself to walk ten paces before I let myself stop to rest and counting these out loud. I thought I might pass out on the path so I tried to walk wherever there was more softness underfoot, a little leaf mould, moss, even grass, and not to walk on rocks, so that if I did fall over I'd have a softer landing.

When I did finally reach the hostel at Roncesvalles, several people immediately came to help me, and someone phoned a doctor. I could hardly speak, by this point, and a kind couple helped me to eat some food and someone else gave me pills for my headache. The doctor thought it was altitude sickness. Altitude sickness supposedly strikes at 8,000 feet (2,500 metres). The highest point of this day's walk had been 4,719 feet (1,430 metres). But I should have realized, since I'd had altitude sickness before at this height. It all suddenly made sense: the confusion and stumbling, the headache, the stupid decision not to let anyone help me.

In my previous mixed-state episode, when I had climbed Kilimanjaro, I had got altitude sickness very badly, with vomiting and headaches and hallucinations (I thought huge banks of snow were white grand pianos), but had refused to come down until I'd reached the peak. I am incautious with altitude, always going higher, faster and further than I should.

Each of the first few days was exhausting. I was walking to my limit and I took Samuel Beckett's line as my mantra: *I can't go on, I'll go on. I can't go on, I'll go on.* On the second or third day, I collapsed on the path, at a bend. I could hear cyclists coming. I hoped they'd be able to stop in time, but I couldn't move out of their way. I remember trying to shout out something, but they couldn't hear because they were yelling and whooping to each other; they were young, energetic, hugely enjoying themselves. They swerved around me, swore at me and swept on without stopping to ask if I was okay. I don't blame them: that state of vigour finds it hard to comprehend weakness, as strength can sometimes fail to understand vulnerability. They probably thought I'd just chosen to stop in a stupid place.

Of course, the Camino is fascinating culturally, spiritually, socially, physically. But it was an ordeal to me, an endurance test. Reading the poems which my friends had given me was the single best part of each day and I could lose myself for an hour or so. I read a Borges poem, 'The Art of Poetry', in Larrasoaña, sitting on a low branch of a tree by a river which flows under a medieval arch. Under the tree, buried among the roots, was an almost completely hidden horseshoe, and it felt like seeing luck itself, almost buried but still glimpsable. The poem recalls Ulysses weeping when he saw Ithaca again, and it made me recall my own Ithaca of art – my work, my words – and I found it unbearable to think about anything I had ever written or ever would. More widely, I was finding my past an anthology of nasty memories; instead of dog-roses, lilies, violets and love-in-a-mist, 'Here,' says remembrance, 'take this,' and sticks me thistles, nettles and brambles, poison ivy and hogweed. No rosemary and too much rue. *Remember to forget*, my footsteps seemed to say, until, after a while, I might even forget to remember and the present tense would spring up, leafy and laughing.

The nights were worse than the days because I had terrible night-mares which waited in the mattresses like fleas. The accommodation in almost all the hostels was in dormitories, with no privacy what-soever, and I knew I was disturbing people around me with my disturbed sleep. One time I woke up screaming and woke everyone else and, although people were kind, I felt embarrassed at leaking my tears and nightmares out all over the place.

I can't tell you much about the Camino itself: I hardly remember much of the actuality of it. It was more prayer than journey, a prayer studded with poems and lit with little kindnesses like candles on the way. A gentle old man offered to carry my rucksack up one particu-larly steep hill. People everywhere seemed to read my face like an open book, and several strangers told me point blank that I needed to learn to accept offers of help, said it was clear I was struggling badly and needed to ask less of myself, that I must realize that I needed to stop. But, from when I was very young, I have felt that I must look after myself in order to be safe. Also, I don't have an off-switch and my will to do this journey was greater than the weakness which undermined me. If willpower has a negative aspect, this is it. I was doing something which was foolhardy: that toughness and hardiness which comes from foolishness rather than wisdom.

I walked with a mixture of suffering and dogged determination, having to endure the ordeal which I had set myself. Loneliness shrieked like the wind around rocks on high passes. I've never longed more for a kind friend beside me, and I felt like the poet of 'The Seafarer', far out to sea, feeling the hardship of being without companion or comfort or consolation yet wanting – yearning – to roam the sea, alone.

Lonely but always surrounded by people: it was the worst of both worlds. Little even made me smile, although the graffiti along the Camino is priceless, especially the thoughts written, etched, chalked or sprayed along the way. (One pilgrim had left a note in pencil, blunt and comic, saying that the only problem with the Camino was that he'd gone seven days without being able to masturbate.)

In a town called Lorca, I read Lorca's essay 'Theory and Play of the Duende', about the surging force which makes real art: 'The roads where one searches for God are known . . . [but] seeking the *duende*, there is neither map nor discipline. We only know it burns the blood . . . that it exhausts, rejects all the sweet geometry we understand, that it shatters styles.'

No church, no matter how grand, neither the cathedral of Burgos nor of León, was as beautiful to me as one ruined hermitage. Dedicated to St Michael, between Villatuerta and Estella, it was completely empty yet absolutely full of prayers, written on scraps of paper: fluttering, forlorn, whispering, weeping, imploring prayers. Hundreds and hundreds of them were written on the back of biscuit wrappers, on pages torn from journals, on old cartons, on the back of receipts; all hand-written, simple prayers from pilgrims, unique and – surely – blessed. St Michael defends and spares, Lorca had written. So I asked for defence against depression.

At the Fuente de Irache, the drinking fountain flows not with water but with wine, and so, in a metaphorical sense, did the fountains of hospitality along the way. Many hostels are run by volunteers, called *hospitaleros* or *hospitaleras*, who look after the pilgrims. (Since everyone is called a pilgrim, no distinction is made over which religion someone follows, or whether they believe in any kind of god at all.) The *hospitalero* job is vital, not only to create practical lodgings but also to make a one-night oasis of kindness for pilgrims, a wellspring in the desert.

One day's walk included a twelve-kilometre stage with no shade, no village and nowhere to stop, and I was walking in 36-degree heat. As no one else was daft enough to attempt that particular stretch in that temperature, I was walking completely alone. At one point, feeling that my head might explode with heat, I scuffed a small hole in the earth under a vine, poured some water in and put my head in the damp, shallow hole. After a while, I walked on. Then one of my boots fell apart. The upper simply divorced the sole. Boots that fit properly are crucial on the Camino and I thought I would have to stop walking, find a large town and buy new boots, which worried me, because wearing a new pair of boots is likely to cause blisters. When I reached the next stopping point, Los Arcos, there was a Flemish confraternity of St James, and I went in, crying with relief, exhaustion, sadness and physical discomfort. They saw my boots and tutted sympathetically. One of the Brothers of the Order looked at my feet, thought for a moment and told me to wait. He left, and came back with a pair of boots which another pilgrim had donated a few days before. They say that 'the Camino provides': you will be given what you need. These boots not only fitted but they were Merrell boots – really good-quality walking boots – and I would go on to do the rest of the journey wearing them. With not one blister.

Even with the new boots in my hands, I was still crying. The woman at the reception desk looked at me kindly and asked what was *really* wrong.

– I've been very ill, I said.

– Very up and down? she asked.

It must have been written all over my face. She gave me a room of my own, and the people who ran the hostel called me La Inferma (the ill one) and treated me with real sweetness. There are things you can do in a room of one's own, and only one of them is writing. I appreciated that probably more than the *hospitaleros* would have done if they'd known.

One day, I heard a bell tolling over fifty times, a weeping, dying toll. I read Rilke's poem 'Let This Darkness be a Bell Tower', and felt as if it had been written for this state of mind I was in:

> *What is it like, such intensity of pain?*
> *If the drink is bitter, turn yourself to wine.*

The Way is both the literal path, signposted with shells, but your Way is also metaphoric: your manner, your habit, your practice. I tried to see the ethics of the Camino as akin to the fairy-tale ethic of being on the path. Keep going; be observant; be kind; be generous; trust that the Way will provide; know that there is only *now*.

I read a page of quotes from Homer one day and didn't know who to pass it on to. The hostel where I stayed that night was small, and very few people understood English. But there was one man who, although I hadn't spoken to him directly, was clearly English. I went up to him.

– Sorry, I said, I know this is a bit odd. But do you want a page of lines from Homer?

He spluttered.

– It's odder than you think, he said. I'm a classics teacher.

And he began quoting me the original ancient Greek.

At a town called Viana, I experienced a biblical hospitality. I was so exhausted when I got to the hostel that the *hospitaleros* told me later I'd gone completely white and collapsed into a chair which they'd rapidly pulled up for me. They gave me water. One of them knelt down in front of me. She took off my boots and peeled off my socks. She brought a bowl of water and a towel, and she gently washed my feet. And I cried. The priest at Santa Maria Cathedral in Viana came to the hostel in the evening and asked us about our reasons for doing the pilgrimage. I was too choked to answer in English. Saying it in Spanish kept a little distance between myself and the words.

– It's a prayer to get well.

– God will answer it.

– I don't believe in God.

– That doesn't matter.

A few days later, when I reached a hostel, as usual – as bloody usual – on the edge of all forms of exhaustion, the *hospitalero*, within five minutes, took me aside.

– Is there some medication you're supposed to be taking which you're not? he asked quietly.

Whoops.

Many of the characters I met on the Camino seemed to have stepped out of the realm of stories. A Frenchman, Roland, called himself (and looked like) a clown; he reminded me of Touchstone, and his speciality was finding four-leafed clovers everywhere. The one person I met coming the 'wrong' way was a conman, insistent that he talked to me and walked with me. All my instincts were jangling.

– I walk alone, I said.

He pursued me. A Catholic friend of mine had very much wanted me to walk with a rosary and, at this point, I saw its immediate protective power: I took it out and pushed it towards him.

– I walk with God, I said, almost hissing.

Then he left me alone.

Within three days of starting the Camino, I had bought a phone and called my doctor and also a few friends. Within nine days I'd begun drinking a few beers at the end of the day. Within ten, I'd bought tobacco. But I was still holding out on antidepressants. I walked and prayed and read and prayed and walked. Walking alone, I often had the feeling that someone was walking just a few steps behind me, and it was a kind, protective presence. Apparently, many other people have felt the same, and some of them call it God.

I saw a man in a religious procession with his hair in tufts of singed swathes. There was zealotry in his face – something medieval about him. A woman sat knitting in a church porch one afternoon. She was ancient and unearthly, like a legendary eternal attendant: her only activities were to knit and to switch the lights on in the church if a pilgrim visited. I stayed a night in a hermitage off the main path, and one of the few others staying was a young Italian guy who was covered in religious tattoos, including a crown of thorns and an enormous face of the suffering Christ. He planned to walk the last hundred kilometres in bare feet because, he said, without pain there was no pilgrimage. He was tattooing his soul as well as his body. In one of the hostels, an ancient and frail woman, clearly disturbed and very confused, was putting on a pair of knickers which looked like mine. Sure enough, when I looked for my own, they had vanished. Outside in the courtyard, a man was painting the old buildings, with their storks' nests and bells, using coffee granules and a tiny drop of water as his paint.

One morning, coming out of a hostel, I couldn't immediately find the way.

– In the mornings, follow your shadow, a passer-by told me.

The enigmatic beauty of that line made me cry. (Predictably.) He looked at me gently and said with real feeling:

– *Buen Camino.*

– Thank you, I said, and *buen Camino* in your life, too.

For the Camino is both footpath and metaphor for one's life.

I met a Swedish journalist who was clever and funny and kind and was walking even though blisters and sores were bleeding right through her socks and her toes were crumpled, blackened bruises and she limped and winced with pain at every step. We stayed together several nights, and one of the many poems I gave her was Mary Oliver's poem 'Wild Geese'.

The soles of my feet hurt constantly, hammered thousands of times a day by sharp little stones. If I walked to the point of exhaustion, I'd get very low because I was so physically tired. If I didn't walk to the point of exhaustion, I started thinking about how little I cared about my life. I had thought that walking the Camino would be a good idea and that if I tried my absolute best I'd be okay, but I was discovering that it was just too hard, and that made me feel disappointed with myself, as well as seriously self-pitying. Buckets of the stuff: revolting self-pity.

To make matters worse, by the halfway point, there were only two nights when I hadn't had nightmares and only one night in the first two weeks when I had slept more than six hours, so I was exhausted from sleeplessness. I walked compulsively, a *fugueur*, needing to keep going in case, if I stopped, I'd never be able to move again. My instinct was (rightly or wrongly) still driving me to view this pilgrimage as a way to get well, to walk the whole hideous illness right out of my system. I felt I had to trust that instinct: 'nor did I look at anything with any other light or guide but the one that burned in my heart,' wrote St John of the Cross, in another of the poems I'd been given, stressing the light of insight, greater than the light of noon.

Indoors, depression coffins the mind. Outdoors, the mind is opened. A pilgrim is, in Spanish, *peregrino* or *peregrina*, because one is crossing the fields: *per* (across) and *ager* (fields). As you walk, you follow the symbol of St James (Sant Iago), the yellow scallop shell, painted on rocks, posts, bins, on tiles or plaques, lined in cement, scrawled, spray-painted or carefully carved. Sometimes the shell morphs into a yellow arrow, and there are thousands upon thousands all along the way, the sign that you are on the right path.

The origin of the shell's association with St James is that a horseman was once saved from drowning by the saint and, emerging from the water, both man and horse were covered in scallops. It is a simple but profound symbol for it is drawn like rays of the rising sun or like the spread fingers of an open hand. It looks like courage, like generosity, like dawn, like the rising of happiness; it is a symbol which protects and vanquishes.

All you need to do to find your way across the whole country is follow these shell-beams, the open hand of an open day. In the caravanserai of days, every day the same yet each entirely distinct, there are no large choices: follow the shells – which also, by taking you on the path from east to west, align you with the two largest signatures of nature, unmissable and utterly reliable: the one the track of the sun each day, the other the path of the Milky Way (also called the River of Heaven), which reflects the Camino, splashed across the sky. This is why Santiago is known as 'de Compostela', for *compostela* comes from *campus* (a field) and *stella* (star). While the capricious shooting stars toss surprising wishes around the night, the constant starlight on the road to Santiago, a *compostela* of the sky, is a constant signature, an affirmed *firma* of faith.

While the destination may be predetermined, yet the manner in which you choose to walk the Way is your choice – like life, of course. The way itself is a surrender to an older order, a Monks' Trod, and yet it is re-determined daily by each individual, and sometimes it takes determination of the grinding kind to walk through both life and the Camino. You follow the path and the path is also recreated within yourself.

One day as I walked I learnt Yeats's 'The Song of Wandering Aengus', its rhythm making the path easier. That evening, among a group of pilgrims, I heard an Irish accent. I felt shy, as awkward as before, but I wanted to give each poem a good home every day.

– Do you want a poem? Dunno if you might want to read it.

The man gave me the widest sort of surprised smile. He had, he said, been longing to read poetry for years, but he had absolutely no idea where to start.

– This would be a good place, I said. Take it. It's by Yeats.

I called my doctor every few days. He was gently but firmly trying to persuade me to go back on antidepressants, but I felt that, if I couldn't come off them here, I'd never be able to. At the same time I felt stupid, hearing myself refusing medicinal help. One day, he commented on the birdsong, which was so loud over the phone that he could hear it hundreds of miles away. I picked up a feather from those singing birds to give him when I was home, and in the meantime it was a talisman to remind me that I was still safe, could still talk to him every now and then, could still feel a line of safety in my hands on the mountain path.

I heard it said that, in the middle section of the Camino, something within you dies. It is a *meseta*, flat and relatively featureless, a hard slog of a week's walk. Halfway through my life, halfway through the road, *mezzo del cammin*, this part was like walking through my illness again. According to some people, it is the most tedious part of the route, but it is filled with millions upon millions of sunflowers in August and no yellow like it. All you can see is acres of yellow and, every day, a huge page of turquoise sky. I was swimming in flowers, daily. But then one day I saw them differently and I thought of van Gogh, whose sunflowers are not laughing but crying, pain-swept with the mad yellow of the overbright light in the mind. I cried for his hurt and humiliation.

The priest at Carrión de los Condes blessed every pilgrim individually, which, with the numbers in the thousands, was a staggering commitment, but people were immensely grateful and he was famous along the Camino for the love and kindness in his eyes.

One evening, I heard a strange sound in a hedge. It was a litter of four starving kittens, hungry and cold, cheeping like baby birds. A woman nearby, who spoke better Spanish than I did, stopped a passing car to ask if the owners of the house knew about the kittens. He was young, pissed and smoking a spliff.

– No, the guy said. It's a holiday home. The mother cat's gone, the kittens'll die.

He scooped them up in an old shirt and put them on the back seat of his car.

– I can't look after them. I've already got four cats. But I'll look after them.

He drove off.

– And he will, said the woman, you could see it in his face.

If you're the kind of man who doesn't like women mentioning periods, you should skip this paragraph. If you're a woman who has walked the Camino, though, you will understand exactly the situation. Getting my period was bad enough, because although about two hundred thousand people walk the Camino every year, there are almost no toilets on the path itself, unless you're passing through a town. Worse, the Camino seems to make women's menstruation impossibly heavy: several women told me they had had the equivalent of two periods in one go – one person I met on the Camino had been hospitalized because her blood loss had been so great. For myself, I couldn't physically walk further.

I stumbled into a hostel, where a young, tough-looking German guy looked at me with something close to contempt for my physical weakness. (I wish that had been the last time I would meet him, but it wasn't to be.) The following day, I took a train for thirty minutes into León, found somewhere to stay and spent an entire day not doing anything much. Except crying. Tediously, endlessly, hopelessly, boringly. That was when I dug my antidepressants out of my bag and started taking them again. I simply couldn't have carried on. The self-pity, for starters, was killing me, and self-pity isn't even *funny*. I hadn't heard a good joke in weeks, and couldn't come up with one. Then I met one.

I ran into a bogus monk. He was Hungarian and said he belonged to an order called the Brotherhood of Mother Teresa. He was obsessive about which supermarkets had the cheapest food and was always trying to get food and lodgings for free. He was completely incurious about anyone else and seemed entirely unconcerned with any spiritual aspect of the Camino. He complained about sleeping in the dormitories 'with people snoring and –' he broke off and made farting sounds with his lips: 'And doing pee-pee. I don't like it.' He piqued my curiosity, because I was fairly sure he was not for real. One day, we happened to check into a hostel at the same time. He told me he had had a massage the previous night – which, on the Camino, was not necessarily the monkish impropriety it might seem, and many hostels offer massages to pilgrims. But then he leant towards me, lowered his voice and said suggestively: 'And then I gave two ladies a massage. Hey?'

His English was pretty good, but when I asked him why he had wanted to become a monk, he didn't know the word. 'What is this word "monk"?' Learning any new language, one learns early the vocabulary for one's own job or vocation. That he knew 'massage' and not 'monk' said it all. Two young Czech women had clocked him by instinct alone.

– Weird man. Fake-monk, said one, shaking her head.

– Look at his eyes. *Whoooeer.*

Their light-hearted grimaces made me giggle for the first time on the Camino, and I was sorry that they were walking so much faster than me and I probably wouldn't ever catch up with them. Later, I met a young English guy who had an infinitely foilable plan to become a monk. He said the Hungarian was fake and he knew why: he could tell from the way the Hungarian wore the cords around his waist.

– He didn't tie his *knots* properly.

The English guy, incidentally, went on to meet a woman on the Camino, fell in love and instantly revoked all his monkish plans. (Bless.)

By this point, I was two thirds through the journey. I'd gone back to baccy, beer and pills and was phoning my friends fairly regularly. One friend of mine decided to come and meet me in Santiago, my longed-for destination. For the first time on the Camino, I felt a real, if momentary, sense of happiness.

I spent a night in the hostel run by the English confraternity of St James at Rabanal del Camino. They organized afternoon tea for the pilgrims and checked everyone for bedbugs. It seemed to be the only hostel that deliberately woke everyone up in the morning and got them out of bed (by playing Vivaldi at full volume). It was also the only hostel to have worked out how not to run out of toilet paper. It was nannying, good-hearted, bossy and hilarious.

At that hostel, I met a young English guy, a student at Cambridge, while we washed our socks at the laundry sinks. He was, he said, trying to learn to be happy.

– How do you do that? I asked: I really, really want to know. I've been a bit crap at being happy recently.

His answers were those of a sweet teenage sage.

– Just four things, he said: Live in the present moment. Have no expectations. And accept yourself and others, accept all your feelings. Feel gratitude for everything which happens.

I thought I was rubbish at all of those things.

– Do you ever read poetry? I asked.

– I'd love to, but I'm an engineer. I'm not *allowed* to, if you know what I mean.

I gave him the poem I'd read the previous day, Rumi's 'The Guest House', perfect for our conversation in this guest house and also for its subject of acceptance:

> *This being human is a guest house.*
> *Every morning a new arrival.*
>
> *A joy, a depression, a meanness,*
> *some momentary awareness comes*
> *as an unexpected visitor.*

. . .

Be grateful for whoever comes,
because each has been sent
as a guide from beyond.

As I walked, I began to feel that at least I would be able to finish the Camino; and I was desperate to meet my friend in Santiago. I also felt for the first time that it was not such a stupid idea to do this walk, after all; to have tried to leave illness behind, to undertake a poem-strewn practice of parting, to break the hold of depression's paralysis. I was also getting physically stronger each day and, thinking back to the beginning of the walk, I was amazed at the difference.

For several days, I walked with a seven-foot truck driver from Denmark who wore fluorescent pink and green clothes and piled pipe-cleaners in her bright blonde hair. She was a walking anti-depressant and seemed a total stranger to sadness. I gave her a poem by ee cummings, one which splashes its infinite blessing for the stout joy of the green world and, to my shock, she broke down in tears for its beauty and told me some of the secret stories of her heart. A friend of mine had given me Rumi's 'The Force of Friendship', which includes the lines 'Anyone who feeds on majesty/ becomes eloquent,' and I gave her that poem, too, because she walked in majesty and talked in majesty and, even when she wept, she wept in majesty.

I tried to learn from the splendour of her strength. Her energy was infectious and vitalizing; her spirit was stupendous. But she was running out of time and had to break off the Camino and go home to her children. I walked on alone, missing her sorely but holding to what I'd felt in the dawns we had seen together, each day's sun a giant apple, slowly ripening over the day.

But nothing comes simple and I knew I was still far from well. It disappointed me bitterly to know that my idea had not worked, that even walking across Spain I could not outpace depression, I could not outwalk it. 'The meaning is in the waiting,' writes R. S. Thomas, and I had to hold on to someone else's wisdom with a patience which is not naturally mine.

Depression still hung in shadows, it gurned in my solitude, it waylaid me if anything difficult happened. And, of course, something difficult did happen. I had a horrible moment when a group of pilgrims had deliberately pushed me out of their way to get into a crowded hostel with a limited number of beds. I was disproportionately upset and tried to get my place back in the queue. The contemptuous young German man I had met before was there. He had seen me move ahead but had not seen the group jostle me out of the way. Suddenly, he sheered round on me, screaming and berserk.

— *I know you, I've seen you on the Camino, I saw you nearly faint on two different days, there is no way, no fucking way, you have walked this,* he said.

His face was six inches from mine, livid with a self-righteous hatred and snarling with the particular contempt that strong people can feel for the weak or weakened.

— *I know you haven't done this on your own. I've seen you crawl.*

At this point he started shrieking.

— *You must have fucking cheated, you must have caught fucking buses and trains and taxis and FUCK knows what else . . .*

I was trembling but furious, and determined to stand my ground. I hate being bullied.

— *Who are you, the Camino fucking Gestapo?* I wanted to say but didn't. I dredged up a residue of grace.

— Yes, I caught a train for thirty minutes on one day. And yes,

I've been ill. And yes, apart from that one day, I have walked every step of the Camino. And I wish you a *buen Camino*.

And then I walked away, but I was shaking uncontrollably. I went into a café, and the barman gave me a cigarette and a glass of water and asked if he could help. I couldn't eat. I could only walk, sick, trembling, angry and frightened that I would re-meet the German guy, because one of the features of the Camino is that one re-meets many people along the way. I walked till late that evening, bought and smoked a packet of cigarettes, rested a few hours and began walking again at 3 a.m. In twenty-four hours, I walked thirty-six kilometres, almost all of it overnight, to outwalk him, to get a day ahead. When I walked in the dark I had often seen shooting stars and, during the small hours of that night, I saw seventeen of them and made seventeen wishes (all for the same thing).

In the morning, to my absolute delight, I re-met the two young Czech women who'd made me giggle. They were sitting at a café having a late breakfast, high on coffee and sunshine and croissants. There was something about their simple, straightforward appetite for life which I adored: an appetite for language, beer, people, knowledge, food and ice cream – always ice cream.

I told them about the screaming German.

– What a *wanker*, one said, bluntly.

– Walk with us. We missed you, we were just talking about you, we were hoping we'd see you again, walk with us.

So all the last few days of the Camino I spent with them, eating, drinking and making merry. They were enjoying their Camino as much as I wasn't. They were as unwilling to reach Santiago as I was keen, but since they could walk about twice as fast as I could, their unwillingness slowed them down to the speed of my willingness and it was an ideal pace for us all. We slept out one night, and I read them lines from St Francis of Assisi's 'Canticle of the Creatures', addressed to 'Brother Sun . . . Sister Moon . . . Sister Water and Brother Fire, through whom You light the night; and he is beautiful and playful and robust and strong'. As they were themselves.

We fell in with a French-Canadian social worker, and the three of them decided to take off their boots and walk barefoot the last six kilometres. They asked me if I'd do the same, and the idea made me laugh out loud. The Camino had forced me to my limit, and burning my feet on boiling tarmac in a Spanish heatwave was just not part of my plan.

Bagpipes played us in to Santiago and we got lost fifty metres before the cathedral. When we finally found it, we went together to the Pilgrim's Mass, watched the vast censer swing, and said goodbye. I was sorry to see them go, but their plan was to walk on to Finisterre, and mine was to get drunk with my friend. When I saw her at the airport, I cried with gratitude and relief and all I could say for an hour and a half was 'Thank fuck it's over.' The ordeal had been endured; all my stumbling, exhausted, aghast month was done.

We spent five days talking, eating, drinking, smoking and sleeping.

– We're surrounded, she said at one point, by unemployed angels.

I desperately wanted to go home: everything in me was yearning for my Ithaca, my cottage, my own patch of garden, my friends, my cats, my woodstove. But I had promised to go to Australia for my book's publication.

I remember little of the trip, except conversations with a few writers and, most importantly, one of my editors, kind and erudite, who saw how fragile I was. Mostly, though, I stayed in bed in my hotel room, getting out only to do talks or for specific interviews or meetings. It seemed a terrible waste of a trip, but I was keening with nostalgia, the aching longing for home. As far from home as it is possible to be, I was horribly homesick. I called the trip short and changed my flights so I could go home sooner. But, in the meantime, it was only in Australia, at that enormous geographical distance from the Camino, that I really began to get a sense of perspective on what 'pilgrimage' really means.

Pilgrimage is an ancient form of travelling for healing, when 'travelling' kept its etymological roots of 'travail' – it is a suffering cure. It is an ordeal to be endured. Perhaps this seems counterintuitive, for illness craves comfort, ease, tranquillity and gentleness, while pilgrimage shoves you into hardship and struggle. Yet to have survived an ordeal makes one feel strong. The relief which comes when the journey is over is more precious for the difficulties of the road, as drinking saltwater makes sweetwater more craved.

There is an automatic lift in the spirits when a difficult time is over, and it reminded me of that kids' game of standing in a doorway, pressing your hands outwards against the door posts for a minute, then walking away and feeling your hands rise on their own. So my spirits seemed to lift of their own accord once I'd finished the punishing pilgrimage. Day after day, I had driven myself onwards, weighed down with a rucksack full of psychological rocks, carrying almost more than I could bear and then, suddenly, in a blink, I could put it down and the lightness streamed through me, weightless in sunlight and I – Heidi.

There is more, though, in the relationship between Path and Pilgrim. The harder I had found walking the Camino, the more I had to mirror it in myself, forced to find rocks of determination to counter the stony paths. I had to become the path, so when it led uphill in a gruelling ascent, I needed to find an equally steep tangent rising within me. In 36-degree heat, I had to match the burning sun on the burning road with my own fire. My obdurate perseverance had to be as relentless as the hours and days trudging through the *meseta*.

The path is laid within us – while we are also inlaid into the path. All the pilgrims who have ever walked the Camino have created it of themselves; our feet have made the paths, our hands have touched the rocks, our boots have carved the holloways deeper into the earth. How much does the pilgrim make the path and the path the pilgrim? It's like Flann O'Brien's story of the postman and his bicycle, which over the years swap molecules in the friction of their journeying. How much of the bicycle is made of postman, or the postman made of bicycle?

A pilgrimage is also curative in creating a pause in one's life, a hiatus, a time when one is exempt from one's own familiar days. It offers an alibi-time, breaking patterns and habits. It gives sickness a chance either to slink away or be held in remission or abeyance. It is a *temenos*, a sacred space, not in place but in time, a set-aside time in which the ordinary is suspended and each day is a holy-day.

On a pilgrimage, the Way heals and so does the Destination. But where exactly is the destination? They say it is Santiago or Finis-terre but, for me, my deepest destination was home. I was in Australia when I fully realized this, right on the other side of the world. My homesickness was not created by the distance so much as symbolized by it.

We are, all of us, on the 'Hero's Journey', in the term popularized by mythologist Joseph Campbell. It is an ancient story and a universal one, a public myth and an individual narrative. The hero – he or she – must both leave and return and, sometimes, the homecoming is more important than the leaving. I had 'left' myself, psychologically, in a terrible withdrawal from sanity, and then I'd physically withdrawn to walk the Camino, so I needed to return, to come home to myself in all senses.

I flew back, stopping a night with my nephews, and found that my Camino was to be book-ended by them when the elder one said he wanted to spend a few days with me. So we returned to my house together. He delights me with the clarity and fierceness of his insight, the gentleness of his nature and the depth of his soul. Having him to stay is like having a dolphin in the house. Because I'd come home earlier than planned, no one was expecting me and I had no commitments or obligations. They were days of grace.

And, in these days of grace, I finally began to know that my month-long walking prayer had been answered; the Camino reconstituted me, but it was only afterwards that I could really feel it.

People who were made to learn poetry at school often speak of how, although they might have resented it at the time, sometimes, many years later, it yields its garlands of flowers. After I'd finished the Camino, the poems I had taken with me were flowering ever more abundantly inside me, my own personal anthology never so beautiful. (An 'anthology' is, etymologically, a garland of flowers.)

One friend of mine had given me Rumi's 'In Baghdad, Dreaming of Cairo: In Cairo, Dreaming of Baghdad'. It hints at the sweetest wisdom:

> *Either this deep desire of mine*
> *will be found on this journey,*
> *or when I get back home!*

> *It may be that the satisfaction I need*
> *depends on my going away, so that when I've gone*
> *and come back, I'll find it at home.*

In homecoming, my body, too, was happy. After the fire, how healing is water. The soles of my feet had hurt for hundreds of hours; they had become swollen with heat, and now they rested cool on fresh grass in my garden. After the thirst and heat of the Camino, I could lean my face against damp, dark moss, and I drank glass after glass of clear, cold water. After weeks of shared showers, insufficient hot water and skimpy little cardboard squares of travel towels, now I had deep baths, with proper-sized towels and, afterwards, my favourite dressing gown. I had the luxury of shady solitude, feeling how priceless is privacy after knowing that your body, awake or asleep, night and day without let-up, can be under the gaze of strangers.

The chancey nature of life on the road was over and I cherished the certainties of home. On the Camino, you don't know where you will sleep each night, but back home is the simplest calm, the humble benediction of one's own bed.

When I was ill before the Camino I had at times felt trapped at home, as if it were an echo-chamber for my psyche and would replay to me my own mind's shriek, ape me the shape of my madness. Homecoming now, I knew it gentle and gentling, newly seen and known, newly and familiarly beloved. Moment by moment, I could feel the consolation of home, my own habitat surrounding me, the intimate miniature world, handmade and tender, the tended home which tends in turn.

Homecoming meant being with my friends, too. When I was ill, my friends understood that 'I' was not 'myself' and they held to their knowledge of the person they previously knew me to be. On the Camino, for the most part, I had hidden, a gaunt ghost in my own days. For everyone on the Camino, one's 'self' is peculiarly unanchored from its past. It can be hard to be a serial stranger to others and, walking ill, the dislocation was doubled: no one knew me, and I wasn't myself anyway. I was unhomed even from my own selfhood, homeless in my mind, but coming home I could feel myself suddenly sturdy in the eyes of friends, my character leaping back like a dog wagging its tail when, after weeks of separation, it eventually hears its own name called.

If this whole year's episode began with falling down a rabbit hole and continued through the dark underworld of suicidality, it ended with a sense of coming up into daylight, small but alive. It would prove to be some months before I was back to my full strength, but this was undeniably the start of wellness.

On the Camino, I had been spent utterly, emptied, dried, withered to nothing, but back home, at the end of it all, I felt a refreshment of sheer water. I felt daybright and eager, my prayers answered in a sweep of benevolence, a superlative generosity of pure largesse, pouring easy and abundant as endless liquid arpeggios. I felt like a small spring on a mountainside, the source of the Wye, water spilling up again and again within me, constantly innerly replenished, liquid life returning, life upwelling in unstoppable wellness.

– How are you? a friend asked me.

– I'm fine. Really *fine*.

I've never said it with such feeling. Fine. 'Fine' meaning 'well'. Up from the good earth, a wellspring of fine water. Fine as a shining field of sunflowers at dawn. Fine as a field of stars in a midnight sky.

ARTIST-ASSASSIN

Poems

Getting My Bearings

When sight is condensed to starlight
Quick to eternity

When mind has thrown its anchor
Back to a raging sea

When the rudder has sheered away in my hands
The boat a stormwracked wreck

And my sails lie in tatters
Mast splintered across the deck

Then reeling round its compass points
Psyche's reason undone

Before behind within and down
Shakespeare Hopkins Donne

I'm steering by the poets now
I'm steering by their song.

Out of Order

At two in the morning
I emailed my friends
Asking if I'd left my hat at theirs
With an urgency previously reserved
For an only-apparently greater loss
An appalled finding:
I find that I have lost
My reason, logic, and – once –
My words.
There, I've said it, as I said it aloud
To myself, on my knees in my study.
Terrified of losing my notebooks
I mark them with my address
Check frantic in my bag every minute or less.
My friend's cancer-scare
I was with her there
In the hallways of the hospital
'This is where I left her.
Can you tell me where
She is?'
'Are you the patient?' an orderly asked
Three times and
Three times I denied it, then
I got the giggles disorderly
At the comedy of loss.

I have lost my mind
My words

My friend
My notebook
And my hat
In no particular order.

Giddy

(for Marg)

Happiness also fathoms things.
My giddy friend plays
Jove, the bringer of jollity,
A one-goddess ode to joy,
She is all the world giggling,
Gravity in reverse,
Serious about frivolity,
A superfluity of light.

Nocturnal in C Sharp Minor

(for George)

I

There is a fathom of a different kind
Which knows the call of the high seas
Where the siren voices steer
And waves have a resonant frequency with mind
The cadences are sheer
Beguiling.

What sounds like song to the mad
Is a deadly wassail
Composed by suicides past
A ship of drunk poets singing up
The tsunami which shatters them
Alluring.

What looks like madness to the sane
Is a self-bewitching:
Spells of the psyche hurled
On its own waters, crying
For the pitch that will rhyme them
Enchanting.

The howling causes
Fractured chords
The devil's interval
Augmented fourth

From crest to gulf
From eros to thanatos
From music to madness
From poetry to anguish.

II

I am a nocturnal in C sharp minor
At three midnights in one: the day's, the year's and mine.
Midnight's alcohol-saddened third
The winter solstice a frost-sharpened seventh
And the minor key's treachery dominant
Seeking the resolution of a chord
Which has been playing me for years –
When the very word suicide has the sweetest ring
In the inaudible octaves far above and below.
I want to die: the phrase is music
I am not the pianist but the keyboard now
Resounded by every hand which has ever touched me.

Tonight transposes all the sounds across the highest Cs
A pitch too much for me –
I have become part of the siren frequencies
Captivated by the acoustics of the deepest seas.
I am being sounded by the sustained notes
At the furthest fathoms of hearing
The high wires which thrilled Odysseus cry for my reply
Knife in one hand, telephone in the other.

III

If I could call into the night
If someone could outshout the siren voices for me
If they would please pick up the phone.
Please pick up the phone:
The prayer which all of those who've been there know.
I know it's late, I know I'll wake your child
I know you know I wouldn't be ringing
Unless what is ringing in me is a terrifying bell –
I am wrung out – I can find no reason not to –
– I have no reason now.
The phone wires ring.
I don't exist
Between notes
Lost for words
Between books
Unharmonized with life
Between no one and no one,
Unless someone could please
Please pick up the phone
My prayer is answered
I ask: Please
Tie me to the mast
Put wax in my ears
So I cannot hear
These terrible siren voices.

One in Five

One in five in this madness
Go and bloody do it: OD, knives or hanging.
But maybe the statistics count it wrong:
It's not one in five people
But one in five moments
One in five devastations
Will wipe you out.
One in five memories
Will explode you.
One in five stalkers
Will catch you.
Maybe everyone can stay with the living four
If they counted different:
Four hours bearable
Four friends reliable
Four hillsides runnable
Four pianos playable
Four poems writable
Not one life unwritten.

Betrayal

Our dreams betray us
To ourselves,
A fraternity of the unconscious
In the corridors of waking.

Spirals

The quixotic spirals of galaxies call me
Towards everything that shines,
Lightning electrifying the mosaic of the stars.
Night sky the first chiaroscuro,
Dazzling distance:
How light defies the dark
Even if the dark was dictated
Long ago,
Light strikes back,
Thousands of years later.

All my moons are spinning out of true
In galaxies of the human mind
Compelled to mirror the real.
With the moons of Jupiter, by Jove,
I can only see in silver and gold,
The spinning light
Where moons both wax and wane.

Wax itself can wane, Icarus,
You and I know, but not yet,
Let me stay here while
The waning earth
Waiting through winter
Wants candlewax, matches, flame,
Until it gets a spring in its step.

But the wax in my psyche is melting,
My mind can't hold itself,
Turning frantic in its circling
The dial of twelve mad hours without words
Until even Mercury knows his day will pass,
Mercredi, even this Wednesday,
And tomorrow he must play his other part, and guide
Me to a hammock of silver silk,
Psyche spun out and back to the cocoon
Of earth.

Essay

I try it once or twice.
Try it with all the scissors I've used
For the literal cut and paste
Editing thousands of paper strips,
Sharpened text on my bedroom floors
For the last twenty years,
Scissors turned happily book-blunt,
Content on the shelves,
The right kind of essays,
The forays of the human mind
Exploring mountains, Montaigne onwards.

This is a trial of a different kind.
I'm trying it out with a Stanley knife,
The wrong kind of sharp,
Implorer not explorer,
A literal essay
Best edited round
Into metaphor.

Because It Snowed on January 18th

A little bird died in the night
Instead of me.
The snowfall which cancelled my voice of reason
And put the cat's-paw in my head
Froze the treecreeper's mind
To reckless and suicidal behaviour
Dropping like a plumb line to the snow
Inviting the cat
Only too happy to accept.

I've shut the cat into the kitchen
With the still bird and the still
Fluttering knife.

Nature's easy, psyche not,
Being both its own
Predator and prey.

Blackbirds

(for Vic)

Blackbirds in London's January pouring their real songs
Into the artificial dawn,
Looking for the trees of Arden
With all their ardent hearts,
Burning from within,
Thinking if they could sing
With more heart, more song,
Then the sun will rise.

Though it is night for hours yet
They sing and burn
And burn and sing
In the false-fire neon
Until the real sun rises
And they burn out into day:
The price of streetlights
Paid in song.

Their hope is a heartbreaking faith
In fake stumps parked
Along pavements which never lead
To the forests, which know no roots
In Arden's earthed, enduring language
Where the birds trust the root-truths of trees
Where, when the real dawn breaks,
It trysts with their unbroken song.

In Reverse

It's the daylight I can't stand.
I can see the dark circles under my eyes,
Reverse moons stitched black
On to the sky of my white face.

By day my hands are purposeless,
Ambling between keyboards, piano and type,
With nothing to play for on either:
By night my fingers feel quick and light.

Hours of daytime stall cold on the floor,
Useless as broken pressure-cookers,
But the night hours are warm and fine
As suns of midsummer.

Night thoughts are lit from the inside,
Candling the living work
Of the kindest poets who revealed most truly
World-mind turned inside out.

Their work is awake, long after they've gone,
Awake and speaking in my night
When – with relief – no one else is here
To mirror to me all that I am not.

One Second

In the distant past
Ten tidy minutes ago,
Checking their watches
They started the car
Not knowing how
In prehistory
Two sad hours ago,
Had I hugged my nephews
One second longer,
I would have come punctual
To the double collision
Of geological time and now
The road punctuated by significance
The failure to read the stop sign
My mind wrecked and reckless
So when I drove across the path
Of their oncoming car
At the fatal crossroad
We were all one bare second away
From something that had already happened.

'The Eye Begins to See'

(see Rilke, 'In a Dark Time')

Poems depend on sight in the dark,
I can only see to write
In the literal night

When this madstruck time began
– Hallucinations enchanting my eyes –
I could see things which were not there

While, driving without looking to see,
I had no regard for what was there
Real as hard metal.

And then my real vision fogged
My left eye could not see the irreal presence
Of some protecting angel

Who measured the distance by which I missed
And made a better judgement than mine
Cast a mist

On half my sight
A spelled-out cast so I cannot judge distance
Out of the question to drive

Staying me to meanings of the righter mind
Found in soft pencil only
And only in the kindness of dark.

The Lonely Letter

I

Lonely as one letter of the alphabet
I walk beyond the snowline of Kili,
A canary for altitude sickness,
I get it violently: quicker than anyone.
My head is an ice palace of crystal pain:
In sick vision, snow is pillows and pianos.
I the inexorable solitude,
A tiny iota divided from other minds.
My idiocy is my implacable will
To go on, against wisdom, against advice.
Because the views from the summit impel me –
Everything here is ice, fire and spirit –
Because the mountains become me
And I can lose myself
Because I can see worlds
And I am unlonely
Because on the top I cannot feel
The peopled isolation of the valleys.

II

If the unlinked climber sleeps
One night on Cader Idris
They wake either mad or a poet
(Or both, poets always reply.)
But the obliterated letter losing sight

Of other eyes knows the third choice
Where the path is a hairpin turn –
Annihilation –
Striking a cliff of fall
Filed away by suicides-future
Like a grid reference:
That's a likely site.
Now is no time to risk it:
Cader is come to me: Kili in my mind.
The snowline has slipped, it
Pillows my voice to a monotone,
Freezes the fingers of friendships,
Ices the keys of the piano
To the unletterable I.

The Price of Argon

(for Iain)

I can feel words with my fingers,
Consonantal cutting rhymes of rock
Chime clean with carabiners
Connecting ropes of thought,
The cadences of vowel slides
Smooth or taut: snow elides
To hollow
While my temples – of Apollo –
Are hammered through with nails
No rhythm except pain.

Why would you climb the human mind?
Not just because it is there
But because all climbers dare the air
Where it is thinnest,
Aware its gases still include dreams.

Too little oxygen to survive,
The body stints its appetite and eats itself,
Anorexia of the heights,
Obsessing every ounce of carried weight,
I can barely drag the whiteness
Of a page to write
Of either the ethereal mind
Or the freighted body.
Climbers call it the death zone,

When they raid it for the summits
For the views – my god –
The vision.

Out on the earthstruck mountain
The head must not mind hurting itself
Skystruck how the price of argon
Has risen to what cost?
All that you possess including – possibly –
Your life.

Argon, the inert gas, is associated not only with inertia but with reverie.

The Traverse

'Make it a short pitch,' I said:
'More accidents happen on the way down.'
So the lead climber was just below me, holding the rope safe,
But in a sudden avalanche he had to swerve away:
The line dangled uselessly,
My mind swinging,
My descent unsecured,
His voice too far to reach me.

I had a choice on the bare rock:
The dutiful
Waiting
Or the beautiful
Traverse –
Truer –
To me –
In a night now voiced with stars.

The utterly speaking part is uttered alone,
The traverse between writer and reader,
Between pencil and page,
Between word and root,
Between language and speech,
Between silence and song,
The sweet and dangerous interval
Between voices.

Parallel Loneliness

(for Ann)

Loneliness is not a word you find in the plural
Lonelinesses would give the lie
To its bound solitude.
Loneliness is the marches,
The no-man's-land between countries:
Loneliness is the marked mind,
The invisible geography,
Territory known by others,
Who have been inwritten
By that same cartography,
Leaving us alike
In worlds alone,
Mapping edge to edge
Our parallel loneliness.

But we have a trick up our sleeve
To defy those maps of the mind:
Faster than prayer,
More certain than pills,
A side-splitting, map-tearing *joke*
Told together:
Hold together, my friend,
I'm right by you.

The Fire of Love

It really would be madness now
To love you
Or you, or you, or you,
Though my heart is on fire.

Someone asked me what is it like, this madness?
Like a wildfire fanned by a hurricane,
A quickened quality of flame
Which knows no borders,
No respecter of persons or properness,
Easy to love anyone but insufficient,
For this is an ordinary fire burning extraordinary
In a world too beautiful to leave,
Where each fir needle is fire
Pure water is fire
Ire is fire
Eyes are fire
Enflamed to seeing
In a fine circle of light
These black suns of knowledge
How the pupil blazes through
To the pure circle of the sun.

It would be madness to love you or anyone
Because this love is a need-fire beyond
Burning for the universal
As transcendental as each of us,

Outsunning the sun
With fire and love and hope:
And the pupils of my eyes are learning
A language of purer flame.

Wavelengths

(for Jan)

Everyone is an exquisite device
For reception and transmission
Wired for empathy
Two-way radios alive
To the acoustics of each other

But the extra sensitivity of certain states of mind
Calibrates at a factor of ten
Each gauge read to a further order of magnitude
Picking up the tiniest signals
Or deafened by the shouts of the over-loud

So the self-obsession of a neurotic
Is an unbearable broadcast of blather
The tedium of a self-repeater
Jangles like an advert for advertising
Avoidance or ear plugs the only strategies

I'm trying to tune in to the wisest wavelengths
The voices which speak their kindness in kind
Which find their way into my mind
Because they know fine-tuning
Is an art where to speak is to listen

Even to the unspoken transmission
The catch in the throat, a way of breathing

The eloquence of silence
The voiced pause
Of the unanswered question

Because they are willing to go an extra order
In the magnitude of the heart.

Hospitality

(for Buʒ and Thoby)

Just how far has a hospital taken leave
Of its original senses
Of providing sacred hospitality
On an uncertain stretch of road, the inn,
In those acres of fields, the garden.
The language of care, cariad,
The caritas for those who are strangers to themselves.
Mercury is guardian of hospitality,
On the horizon for lost eyes, a focal point,
A *fuego*, the warmth of 'hearth',
Folding in one warm word heart,
Heat, earth, hear, eat – and the tea
As a child in my grandmother's house
By the stove, bread rising,
The yeast, the wine
Of consecrated trust
That there will always be a welcome
For those suffering hiraeth away
From their own mind's square mile
So everywhere is home, as ungated
As gratitude, as grace.

Cariad (Welsh): 'dear'. Hiraeth (Welsh): 'homesickness'.

Patient Doctoring

Sometimes a doctor must be patient with himself
Holding back the frustration of the desire
To act, intervene, inject, prescribe
Because a patient's description may be more curative
Than a doctor's prescription:
The telling of telling details of a life.

A doctor wants someone up, out of bed, on their feet – of course –
To speed the course of illness.
It is harder to be willing to wait awhile
As the mind takes its own courses
In the paths of its own cures:
The guiding word is *docere*,
Leading someone by the hand through madness
And fine doctoring is a subtle profession
Willing to watch, wait, attend,
Attentive to the quiet admissions
When a doctor's first and greatest skill is to listen.

I shrink from unkindness.
I wane at insensitive remarks.
But a crescent kindness
Kindles me like the moon
Waxing back to its full brightness.
It finds me, moves me:
Injections of reassurance twice a week
Interventions of thoughtfulness

Kindness a force against which even my nightmares weaken.
Fiercer, tougher, willing and wise to the medicine of time.

For the off-kilter mind
Listening is another form of intensive care.
I daresay it would be easier
To commit a patient talking suicide.
Far harder to take the other route
To the roots of this kind of pain
Not sedating suffering
But slowly – patiently – actually
Undoing its terrible hold.

The Question I Would Like to Ask a Shaman Now

Not how to fly.
Not how to hear the messages on the highest hills.
Not how to discern good angels from destroying ones.
Not even how to find the poetry.
But how to get back safe from the night-shade,
Night-vision intact, tucked poems in my rucksack.

If I answered my own question
It is to attend each occluded step
Beware the accidents of descent
Keep a constant vigil
A stern metallic grip
Holding fast to bread and water.

It is not to flinch at the knowledge
I have to climb down lonely as I climbed up
Fabulously alone.
To use each herb-word, each verb-root
Because the only thing which unclouds my solitude
Is language.

It is to find the courage to leave the allure
To return to the softer shore
Of the lovely dayside
The tidy fireside
Clean cups, stocked woodpile,
The written book, completed work.

In Thanks

For the sensitivity and tenderness of many people along the way, too numerous to mention, I offer my poignant appreciation. I drink to all tendernesses.

For those cherished friends who took care of me with enduring loyalty and lit candles in the dark: Ann Clare, Niall Griffiths, Anna Jenkins, Deborah Jones, Nicoletta Laude, George Marshall, Thoby Miller, George Monbiot, Marg Munyard, Eddie Parker, Jan Parker, Andy Scrase, Hannah Scrase, Thea Stein, Buz Thomas, Andy Warren and Vic Worsley.

For being the apple of my eye: David Griffiths and Timothy Griffiths.

For such wise and comradely encouragement, a deep bow to Barry Lopez, Iain McGilchrist and Philip Pullman.

For kindness, intelligence and support far beyond the call of duty, I salute my agent Jessica Woollard and my editor Jack Shoemaker, together with Anna Ridley and Anna Kelly. Thank you with all my heart.

And for the profound skill and care of Dr Leslie: I hope that this book itself stands as my testament of gratitude. It dedicates itself to you.

Printed in the United States
by Baker & Taylor Publisher Services